the body of life

ALSO BY THOMAS HANNA

The End of Tyranny: An Essay on the Possibility of America (1976)

Bodies in Revolt: A Primer in Somatic Thinking (1970)

The Lyrical Existentialists (1963)

The Thought and Art of Albert Camus (1958)

BOOKS EDITED BY THOMAS HANNA

Explorers of Humankind (1979)

The Bergsonian Heritage (1963)

the body of life

Creating New Pathways for Sensory Awareness and Fluid Movement

Thomas Hanna

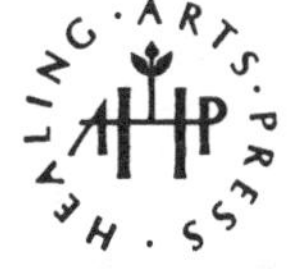

Healing Arts Press
Rochester, Vermont

This book is dedicated to the two men who in their own way taught me to revere the earth:

Albert Camus *Moshe Feldenkrais*

Healing Arts Press
One Park Street
Rochester, Vermont 05767
www.InnerTraditions.com

Healing Arts Press is a division of Inner Traditions International

Note to the reader: This book is intended as an informational guide. The remedies, approaches, and techniques described herein are meant to supplement, and not to be a substitute for, professional medical care or treatment. They should not be used to treat a serious ailment without prior consultation with a qualified healthcare professional.

Library of Congress Cataloging-in-Publication Data
Hanna, Thomas, 1928–
The body of life : creating new pathways for sensory awareness and fluid movement / Thomas Hanna.
p. cm.
Originally published: New York : Knopf, 1980.
Includes bibliographical references and index.
ISBN 978-0-89281-481-7
1. Manipulation (Therapeutics) 2. Mind and body. I. Title.
RM724.H36 1993
615.8'2—dc20 92-47112
CIP

Printed and bound in the United States

12 11 10 9

Drawings by Anita Karl

contents

preface

What is life? is one of the favorite questions of the human race. In times both of crisis and of quietude this question arises as an ultimate attempt to make sense of things. The same question has been answered millions of times and, of course, in a million different ways. This is because there is neither a right answer nor is there a final answer; the question is so broad and so vague that almost any answer will do.

This is not to say that the question is unimportant. There is, perhaps, no question so significant. But the problem is that the question is always wrongly phrased. To ask, What is life? is to treat life as if it were an abstraction, as if this were the same as asking, What is truth? or What is goodness? The question is wrong because life is not an abstraction; it is always something very concrete, for life exists in one form and in one form only: in living bodies. Outside of individual bodies there is no life. Life does not occur except in embodied form, and when we see and experience life, it is always by seeing and experiencing a living body.

When we cease to think about life as an abstraction and begin thinking of it in terms of the specific living bodies in which life exemplifies itself, both the question and the possible answer begin to take on a different meaning. If we rephrase the question correctly and ask, What is the nature of a body that has life? then we can answer the question in a way that makes specific sense. Whatever life may be in abstraction, we know that the way life manifests itself in living bodies is through autonomous *movement.* The living body is a moving body—indeed, it is a constantly moving body. This is the prime trait by which we recognize life and distinguish the "quick" from the "dead."

The movement of a living being is of a unique kind: Living bodies are self-moving; they are individual systems of movement, moving in organized, coordinated, sequential ways. If we are to be precise, we must say that life exists always and everywhere in one characteristic form: as the organized movements of an individual body.

It would, then, seem obvious that to understand life means to understand the ways in which individual beings move. I do not wish to suggest that this suddenly simplifies the question What is life? but it makes it more concrete. A living, moving body is far from being simple, however concrete a fact it may be. It is, as we shall see, a matter of immense complexity and mystery. But at least this concrete way of posing the question gives us something to focus on and analyze.

This book is about life in the concrete sense that all of us know life: in living bodies. It is primarily about the living bodies of human beings, but it is also about the living bodies of all species of animals. The more closely we look at the nature of organized movement in individual bodies, the more it becomes obvious that beneath the veneer of human language and human culture we are far more like our fellow animals than we have ever known or ever dared to admit. It is my conviction that the difference between a healthy, fully functioning amoeba and a healthy, fully functioning man is very slight and that, because they are oblivious to the crucial factor of physiological movement, the working models of psychology, psychotherapy, and medicine are largely inappropriate for understanding human beings.

The identification of life with movement can be carried a step further if we entertain the following possibility: If life means movement and death means nonmovement, then it may be permissible to think that more movement means more life and that less movement means less life. I believe that this is, in fact, the case, and in the first chapters of this work I want to present ample evidence that a diminished capacity for movement is equivalent to diminished life. Conversely, it will be made clear that to enhance the efficiency of bodily movement is to enhance the vitality of human beings in all of their functions, whether physical, mental, or emotional.

These convictions are not so much the product of philosophical speculation as they are that of practical discovery. I work with people who are crippled, paralyzed, or in acute muscular pain, using my hands to teach them to expand the range and efficiency of their bodily movements. I am not a physician who cures; I am an educator who teaches, and in the course of my teaching I have discovered an extraordinary thing: Most adult human beings have very little ability to sense the movements of their own bodies and consequently have little ability to move and control their bodies. The sensorimotor functions at the heart of the human central nervous system are, in the typical adult, atrophied. Except in rare instances the contemporary, urbanized human being reaches adulthood with a sensorimotor system that is only minimally developed, and then, during the remainder of his life, he steadily loses the ability both to sense his body and to move it efficiently.

All of us prefer to think that the growth and maturation of a human individual entails a growth in self-consciousness and self-awareness. Presumably, the great difference of civilized men from their brutish, primitive forebears is in the cultivation of self-awareness. This, however, is not at all the case. In primitive societies the sensorimotor development and the proprioceptive-somesthetic faculties of self-sensing are highly developed. These neural faculties of bodily self-awareness are highly developed for the simple reason that, in primitive environments, survival requires it. But in urbanized man the reverse development occurs; contemporary education and culture are designed to limit and stifle the development of the faculty of self-sensing, so that by the time adulthood is reached, the individual's awareness of his own physiological being is so dulled and obscured that he feels that his consciousness is lodged inside a foreign encasement. The process of acculturation takes the lively self-awareness of the infant and steadily represses it, while at the same time it encourages the development of the exteroceptive senses, so that the final result is someone who is highly aware of the external world and pitifully unaware of the internal world of his own body.

This lack of self-awareness is not a minor matter. It is a major catastrophe for modern society. It is catastrophic because the steady loss of our sensorimotor abilities guarantees that by the time men and women reach middle age, they will most likely discover—always to their surprise—that their vertebrae are distorted and that they have lower-back pains, sciatica, and chronic stiffness and soreness in the neck and shoulders. For another thing, the lack of sensory self-awareness allows unperceived strains and pressures to accumulate over such a long period that strokes, heart attacks, and other physiological breakdowns occur without warning. Lack of self-awareness is not simply a moral problem, it is the major public health problem of contemporary society. Our cultural program is a program of human diminution and destruction, but because culture is as invisible to the acculturated human being as is water to the fish, we cannot see that these breakdowns are not the normal and inevitable results of aging but are the abnormal and preventable results of cultural conditioning. Stated simply, the typical mental and physical diseases of our society are *learned.*

The more closely we look at a living body, the less solid it seems. The solidity is purely illusory. Underneath that stable-appearing shape is a network of ordered movements that are as ceaseless as they are complex. It is this hidden system of movements that we shall explore and attempt to understand. Beneath the level of our verbal, acculturated consciousness is a realm that we are only now beginning to perceive and trace out. I call it the somatic realm—*somatic* because it sees the human being and all living beings not merely in terms of bodily structure but in terms of bodily function, namely, movement.

Only during the last century have we become aware of the somatic realm, and only during the last generation has this realm revealed its avenues of practical application. These avenues are the directions taken by somatic educators, who have succeeded in bringing about human change in ways that had not, up until now, been thought possible.

I particularly want to focus on the practice of Functional Integration, the most effective and clinically specific form of somatic education. Invented by Dr. Moshe Feldenkrais, an Israeli scientist, Functional Integration seems upon first acquaintance to be a kind of magic. What it accomplishes with the human body appears, initially, to be impossible.

Functional Integration is neither magic nor miracle. Instead, it is a straightforward application of the principles of somatic education. A number of case histories are given in this book to illustrate the nature and effects of Functional Integration. Each of these case histories is followed by a discussion of the specific somatic function revealed by the case history.

Finally we will be able to draw certain conclusions that will enable us to understand why these "miracles" can occur to human beings and can do so consistently and predictably. However, first let us take a brief look at this four-dimensional oddity, the soma, and notice how certain universal physical forces have inscribed themselves into the very constitution of living bodies. The somatic realm is as fascinating as it is surprising. Moreover, it offers us a practical understanding of the human being that is, I believe, the harbinger of a new era in human education and medicine.

the body of life

introduction: what is a soma?

The tree of life is immensely large and complex, and we of the human species are one twig on that tree. A twig is not representative of the whole tree but is a very specialized development of it, so that, if we wished to understand the whole tree, we would avoid looking at it from the twig's specialized point of view and choose, instead, that of the roots and trunk.

A twig's-eye view of life is obviously a distortion, yet it is a distortion dear to us all. It is called anthropomorphism —that is, looking at all things from the human point of view. The sapience of *Homo sapiens* has, because of this distortion, had a tattered history. It pleased us to believe that the universe was created for us, even as it seemed obvious that all the stars found their center in us and our earth.

Losing our naïve bent toward anthropomorphizing the

world has been slow and painful, and this bent has blocked the progress of controlled scientific understanding from its beginning. Because all living beings are centers unto themselves, it is quite probable that every living creature, if he were articulate, would look at the tree of life from his own point of view—the oysters would have their version, the algae theirs, and the aardvarks theirs.

It was the twig's point of view that was offended by the results of Charles Darwin's patient and painstaking research. The twig characteristically thought of itself as the center of life—God Himself had ordained it this way, and He completely supported the twig's-eye point of view. Such an attitude does little good for the reputation of either science or God, since neither is committed, traditionally, to a narrow view of things.

Undeniably it was painful to acknowledge that the sun does not go around the earth, but this loss of human pride was, at the same time, the scientific prerequisite for man setting foot on the moon. In just the same fashion, it is painful to share Darwin's viewpoint that the human species is not the model and standard of life but one of its most specialized forms. Darwin dispelled thousands of years of illusions that had blinded us to the fuller nature of our identity with the universe. In a most exact sense, the "science of man" became possible for the first time at the moment when man was removed from the center of the scientific stage. Then, abruptly, we were able to see ourselves in terms of a larger context—in terms of the cosmological, physical, chemical, and biological context out of which all life arose.

It is this broader context that science—in response to Darwin's invitation—has investigated during the century since Darwin. If we look at the atmosphere and the soil, and then at the roots and the trunk, we can discover a vision of ourselves that is considerably less distorted, a vision that attempts to embrace the full context of evidence without excluding parts of it. The research of the past century has fleshed out and confirmed Darwin's broader vision in the fields of genetics, biochemistry, biophysics, ethology, anthropology, neurophysiology, and many others.

The first thing that this broader context tells us is that life entered this world in the form of a body. It is the shape of life that first impresses us. Because it arose out of the physical universe, life took a shape that looked vaguely like any other body of matter. It looked solid just like a physical object; this was because it used a certain number of terrestrial atoms, just as all earth objects do. At first glance, life's body looked like a physical body, but what was radically different was that it did not behave like a simple collection of atoms. It moved independently, it reproduced itself, it selectively exchanged chemicals with its environment, it held together as a single system, and it did many, many other things, as we shall begin discovering.

The body of life that unfolded itself on this earth is, in fact, unlike any other body in the world and must not be confused with the simple physical bodies of the world. To avoid such confusion, it is better to use a more ancient and appropriate word for life's body: That word is *soma* (Greek: σωμα).* In Greek, the word *soma* evolved to

*This is not to be confused with the Vedic word *soma,* which was made popular by Aldous Huxley in his *Brave New World* and referred to a mind-altering drug.

mean "the living body in its wholeness." It is also a term used by biologists to distinguish the full living body of an animal from its chromosomes.

It was the soma that arose from those long-ago tide pools. The shape chosen by life was not simply three-dimensional. The body of life was and is four-dimensional; it has height, depth, width, and time. The soma arose as a system that always strives to achieve stability and balance —a task that takes place in time and is never complete. In its internal functions as well as its external actions, the soma times itself; that is, it measures and coordinates its movements in sequence.

To say that the soma has an element of timing is the same as saying that the soma is not a thing or objective body but, rather, *is a process.* That is another reason for holding to the word *soma* rather than the word *body.* The latter word suggests something that is static and solid. A soma is neither static nor solid; it is changeable and supple and is constantly adapting to its environment.

But to say that the soma is an adaptive process that times its actions is tantamount to saying that it is an integral system. To refer to the process of a billion atoms as "it" is a sure sign that a higher-order synthesis has taken place. Life's soma is a system moving through time, and it is the living system that endures and has identity, despite the fact that during the lifetime of any soma—one-celled or multicelled—all of its "physical" atoms will be replaced countless times. The soma has a synthetic integrity that holds together through time.

Beyond this, to say that the soma is a systemic process is to say that "it" has some central control that is responsible for the whole process. The central, executive control of a neural system—structurally obvious in higher animals—is functionally obvious in the simplest one-celled organisms. An amoeba, for example, has neither skeleton nor muscle nor central nervous system built into its structure; nonetheless, it acts as if it did. It moves and "walks" quite well by extending its boneless pseudopods, planting them and then literally pouring its cytoplasmic self into the new space created by the pseudopods. Such systemic control demonstrates that the *function* of the nervous system existed from the beginning. It required millions of generations and mutations for the neural structure to catch up with the neural function.

The soma is the body of life, and there is nothing else like it. What an extraordinary being life introduced into the world: The soma appeared as a whirling, integrated process of atoms that behaved freely and independently of the rest of the world. More extraordinary than that, the identity of the soma was so strong that its actions *were intended for itself.* The body of life had its *own* interests and its *own* needs, and its constant movement was intended to satisfy those interests and needs. It was the original cybernetic system; that is, it was *self*-guiding.

In the same way that a soma is not a "body," it is equally not a "mind," "spirit," "soul," or any other such human projection. The soma is more than all of the religious and philosophical abstractions that clutter the heads of human beings; it has always been far more than that, from the very beginning. There, within the first cell, the complex secret of life was already spelled out, at least implicitly. It simply took some time, immense aeons of time, for those original secrets to begin to unfold and to structure themselves explicitly in the tree of life. Even as the soma finds its original nature in the physical universe out of which it naturally arose, so will we, as human somas, find our original nature in the primal soma out of which we have arisen.

The soma is not an object, it is a process. In the same way, life is not a "what" but a "how." To understand the soma and its process is to understand the how of life.

It is the shape of life that reveals how much living things are expressions of the universe and its physical laws. These laws—notably the thermodynamic and gravitational laws—sculpture the soma like invisible hands. These hands inevitably mold living matter into a shape that is compact and economical: a round, three-dimensional shape.

The second law of thermodynamics as well as the law of gravity decree that a rounded shape is the most economical way of operating. They decree the same shape for atoms and for solar systems. The rather recent discovery of the molecular structure of genetic inheritance was a spectacular view into the shape of things at the heart of the reproductive system. The DNA molecules that make up the code of genetic information are long chains of building blocks called nucleotides. These nucleotide chains might conceivably stretch out randomly in any direction like a loose rope, but this is not what happens. Instead, the nucleotides form a pair of chains that coil around each other in an elegant, tight spiral. That is the shape of DNA: roundness.

We all know that single living cells tend to be rounded and compact—microscopes show us that. But with an electron microscope we can probe much more deeply into the cell. And at this minute level, we again see the same attempt of living matter to take on the shape of a three-dimensional soma.

For example, the hemoglobin in our red blood corpuscles is a typical protein molecule, built up of chains of amino acids. In the large hemoglobin molecule there are precisely 574 amino acid molecules arranged in 4 chains. We might think that these molecular chains would flair out this way and that, each entangling itself with other organic material in some random manner. However, these long chains twist around one another in an incredibly complex way to form a globular, three-dimensional structure that looks very much like a thick bush. Our bodies contain millions of these hemoglobin bushes, and the astounding fact is that *each one is exactly identical with the other.* This is an example of life's extraordinary stability and order. In the case of our own bodies, the physical laws underlying and controlling matter *shape four hundred million million exactly similar hemoglobin bushes every second, while destroying the same number every second.* This is an example of how life is a stability within an unstable process.

It is the tendency of all life to shape its molecular elements into the three-dimensional shape of a rounded body. This process goes on at the microscopic level of molecules and cells and at the macroscopic level of complex animal bodies. At any level, it is the same somatic process.

Atoms have different shapes, like different pieces of a three-dimensional jigsaw puzzle; they can fit with other atoms only in certain ways. And they "fit" in very concrete, physical ways. Turned a little this way or that, two atoms will not join in forming a molecule; but turned just right, so that this atom's brace of electrons meshes exactly with that one's electrons, and there is suddenly a fit—a "bond." Atoms bond with each other to form larger structures, such as molecules, in somewhat the way that the fingers of one hand mesh with those of the other hand for a tight fit.

The protein chains that make up the prime contents of living bodies all have a three-dimensional shape. They are microscopic somas—protosomas, having a skeleton but no flesh. Some shapes are made to fit with one kind of element; other shapes will fit only with a different jigsaw piece. Different atomic arrangements in the chain make it possible for the protein to pick up, fit into, and interact with very specific elements. Each protein chain is specially arranged to have a certain kind of chemical reaction; it will interact only with certain chemical nutrients, retaining what it needs and ignoring what it doesn't need.

The chemical factory lodged within the tiny body of each living cell is surprisingly simple in its architecture: Every protein chain in the production line is a combination of amino acid residues, which belong to only twenty different chemical species. And these twenty chemical arrangements are found in all living species, from bacteria to man. All of the millions of different species on this planet have been put together from the same common stock of chemical possibilities.

Because life must obey universal physical laws, it always shapes itself into efficient, economical bodies. The cell is certainly compact and well integrated. It can be round like a ball or elongated like a sausage, with many variations in between. But whatever the exact shape, all cells have a somewhat rounded structure neatly contained within a surrounding membrane.

Children love balloons with long ears and a prominent

nose. When they squeeze the two ears, the nose gets bigger. When they squeeze the ears and the nose, the face gets bigger. And when they squeeze the face, the ears and nose get bigger. Parts of the balloon expand and contract, but the contents and the pressure of the balloon never change during the child's squeezing; they remain constant and balanced. The universe, as a whole, conserves its total energy in this way. The energy may go from this place to that, but within the total system it remains the same.

It remains the same, but with one crucial difference: The movement of energy back and forth takes a bit of starch out of the atoms involved; the "free energy" they possessed is leeched out of the atoms in the form of movement and heat, and this heat, once expended into the vast cold of the ether, is lost forever. When atoms spend their free energy, they become quieter. A boulder perched on top of a hill has great energy available for movement, but once it has rolled down to the bottom, it has lost that free energy. It is still, atomically, the same boulder, but its situation has changed. It can regain its former potential energy only if *more* energy is borrowed from elsewhere to roll it back up. On its own, the boulder will never recoup its loss.

All of this is a simplistic way of describing the most fundamental of physical laws: the laws of thermodynamics. The first law says that the total energy of the universe remains constant, just as does the interior of the child's balloon. The second law says that every event in the universe is like a boulder rolling down a hill—the free energy, once expended, cannot be replaced. The universe is gradually losing its punch, and this tendency to run down is called entropy. The third law states that the only way to avoid entropy is for matter to be in a perfectly stable crystalline state at absolute zero—in this case "zero" means absolutely without heat or movement. The third law is an ideal theorem for the overcoming of entropy; it is not, however, a fact. Neither in the universe nor in the laboratory is it possible to create the perfect immobility of zero heat.

It is bothersome, this second law of thermodynamics, for it tells us that the entropy of the universe steadily increases, that the universe is running down, getting slower and cooler as it dissipates its free energy. Looked at closely, entropy is a curious thing: It is the loss of a certain order or arrangement. It takes a certain arrangement of things—like a boulder on top of a mountain—to create the energy for movement and heat; once that arrangement has been abandoned, so has the energy. Rather than being in an orderly arrangement, it falls into disorder, randomly arranged. Upon closer examination, entropy appears to be the universal necessity of physical order declining into randomness, just as the tides of the unstable universe wash back and forth, using up heat.

One of the fundamental characteristics of the living cell is that it has relatively little entropy or randomness; indeed, when cells are dividing or rapidly growing, entropy is reversed. Organisms, from their very beginning, met the second law head on and managed to work with the situation—very efficiently. They did so by the way in which their bodies were arranged: Organic bodies have a most special kind of order, namely, an order that minimizes the loss of order. This organic order is the dynamic "steady state" by which organisms break down their lipids, polysaccharides, and proteins while continually replacing them. The turnover is enormous. It is also complex. Living cells are complex systems, involved in an open exchange with the environment while maintaining a steady internal state.

What the law of entropy teaches us is that order is a form of energy. Thus, life seeks to preserve its cellular order by intricately structured macromolecules that are rich in information and that allow the cell to be self-adjusting.

The organic realm arose as a higher ordering of the inorganic realm—a higher-order synthesis that gathers atoms together into a constantly varying dance. This dance is orderly precisely to the extent that it is complex and unceasing. The history of life is one of increasing order and decreasing entropy—the more complex the dance, the more efficient the system.

Because life arose as a higher-order synthesis of elements, it had to come to terms with the second law. And life's response to the law of entropy is to organize a collection of atoms so that the presumed loss of free energy does not necessarily occur. Chemical forces are arranged in such a way that they fall together into a self-balancing, nuclearlike system. In the living cell everything flows into everything else in a continual sequence of smooth reactions between the cell's many parts. It is an almost frictionless process of such enormous efficiency that it requires only a slight input of outside energy to make the incredible machine run.

According to the laws of thermodynamics and gravitation, the perfectly efficient and economical shape of life is that of a globe. When, in general, we think of somas, we should imagine them as rounded beings enclosed within a membrane.

And when we look at our own bodies, we see the same structural theme: a round, elongated shape within a sack of skin. When we look at other animals, whatever their shape, we can see the abiding shape of the soma just underneath.

On second glance, I realize that my body is not exactly a single body. I could also look at it as a collection of one-celled bodies. It is a soma made up of somas. How can that be? It can be because the tendency of all life is to somaticize itself efficiently, and this is most dramatically displayed at the multicellular level of animal bodies, the Metazoa. The jump from one-celled life to multicelled animal life seems immense until we remember the demands of the second law: A group of single cells will come together in a higher-order synthesis if that synthesis is more efficient and economical.

The second law of thermodynamics is a central factor in the evolution of species. It was the second law that caused the emergence of the first soma, the primal cell, and it was the same law that grouped cells together in such a way that they form a community. A community of cells is a higher ordering of the physical elements of the cells, so that, together, less entropy occurs. And this is what happened with the jump from single-celled bodies to multicelled bodies, namely, the jump from Protozoa to Metazoa on the tree of life. The evidence of this higher order is stamped into every cell. Each cell bears the entire chromosome code of the animal; the cells of complex animals are typically "branded" with the same species identity.

The Metazoa are more efficient in the conservation of energy because they can handle energy more complexly and with more stability. And the more complex the order, the more efficient the biological system—that is the biological rule. The evolution of species is the appearance of ever more subtle and intricate ways of preserving order and energy.

Such considerations may at first seem rather remote from the daily affairs of our lives and our bodies, but they are not. They are vital to an understanding of our lives and bodies. To make this clear, we will look at case histories of typical human beings whose bodies have become inefficient and no longer work well. Something has gone wrong with the way their bodies function. They themselves do not know why this has happened; their physicians, psychiatrists, and psychotherapists do not know. Their ailments are a mystery to everyone. It is our task to clear up the mystery. In doing so, we will discover some extraordinary things about the body of life.

ONE / THE FOUR DIMENSIONS OF THE SOMA

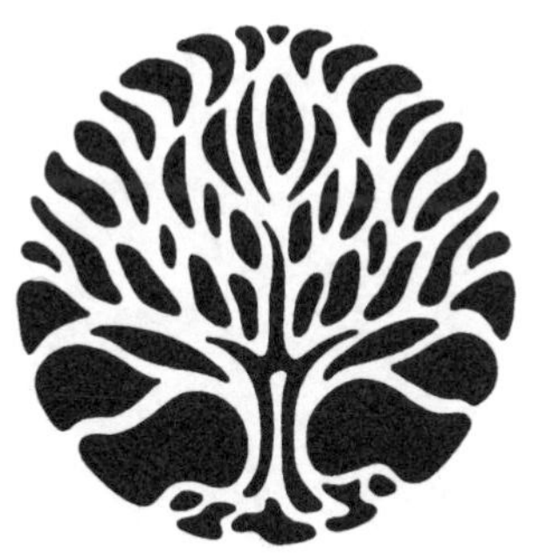

1 / spatial distortions of the living body

SOMATIC RETRACTION

When I saw Pat M. for the first time, he was a man in desperate trouble. For nine months he had been in constant pain, and his face showed it: The eyes were constricted, the mouth was a tight, grimacing line, and the head was locked backward to the right, as if someone were pulling his head from behind. He moved very little and slowly; the least sudden motion caused him to wince from the pain in the right side of his neck and shoulder.

Although he had had occasional pains in his lower back, he had never been aware of any other problems in his body until July of the year before, when he dove into a swimming pool only to discover that the muscles in the right side of his neck suddenly contracted, drawing his head backward in extreme pain. Pat was head of a large, highly successful real estate agency and was on a medical insurance program that allowed him unrestricted clinical diagnosis and treatment.

He was first advised to treat the neck pain by resting, using heat, and taking pain killers. He tried this, but the involuntary contraction of the neck muscles continued unabated. In response to this his physician began a program of drug treatment, using muscle relaxants. This again seemed to make little difference, so the decision was made to put him on tranquilizers, which, he said, left him woozy and made it difficult to perform well in what was an extremely high-pressure job.

The next step was more direct: the use of high-frequency electrical and sonic stimulation to induce the neck muscles to relax. This again proved futile, so it was recommended that he try physical therapy. The therapist put him in a machine that pulled on the head and forcibly stretched the neck muscles. The effect of these treatments was that the neck became even sorer and the head was pulled back more tightly.

Nothing seemed to work, so he was referred from orthopedics to neurology, then to psychiatry, then to other clinics until, as he told me, it seemed as if he had seen over a hundred physicians, who gave him a hundred different clinical opinions, none of which made any difference. So that what I encountered on that April afternoon was a highly successful thirty-eight-year-old executive now wearing a neck brace, heavily sedated with pain killers, and desperately fearful that he was permanently disabled and would be forced to quit working.

I asked him to remove the neck brace and lie down on his back on a padded table. I placed a small pillow under the back of his head and neck to make him comfortable and lifted his knees to place a bolster under them so that they would be slightly raised. Looking at him lying on his back with the head pulled back at an angle and with his shoulders high, I was reminded of the posture of someone who was cringing, like a child who, when frightened, will retract his neck, pulling it down between raised shoulders.

He said he was comfortable now and, being careful not to disturb that comfort, I began to move his body very gently in an effort to see the quality of the muscular tonus in different joints. I should mention that when a person is standing, the general tonus of his musculature is quite high, but when that same person is lying horizontal, no longer resisting the vertical pull of gravity, the musculature will relax. At least it will relax up to a certain point: Lying horizontal, the person will no longer be making voluntary movements of his muscles, but—and this is a crucial point—if there is involuntary contraction of these muscles, one can immediately discover it by gently moving that person's limbs. If, despite the relaxation of all voluntary movement, there is activity in the muscles, then we know that we have discovered patterns of involuntary muscular contraction that are taking place in that individual's body, whether he wishes it or not and whether he knows it or not.

This is exactly what I discovered in Pat's body. I lifted the right leg, bending the knee, and then, with the thigh vertical, began slowly rotating the leg in a small circle. Since Pat was relaxed and not doing anything, one would think that the leg would make a smooth, effortless circle. But this was not the case. As I rotated the leg, it would jerk and resist the movement, veering away from the circular line I was describing. It was as if there was a perverse puppet master inside who had his own ideas about how the leg was to be moved.

I walked around the table and lifted his left leg. When I attempted to rotate it, the same involuntary resistance occurred. Then I lifted his right arm, beginning a slight movement of the shoulder blade. Here the jerking and resistance were much more pronounced, and the shoulder blade was leaden and heavy; I could just barely move it. Then I went to his left arm. As I lifted it, the elbow jerked and fidgeted as if fighting the movement. The shoulder blade was solid and immobile, as if it had been cemented. Softly I touched the right side of the trapezius muscle behind the neck. It was rigidly contracted.

That brief inventory made it clear that there were, in a sense, two persons lying on the table. One person was the self-aware, voluntarily moving Pat, who was now attempting to be totally relaxed; and the other person was an unconscious, involuntarily moving Pat, who acted quite independently. The cause of the trouble was this unconscious, involuntary person. It was he who was cringing, creating a major contraction of the neck, a minor contraction of the lower back, and a general contraction of the shoulder and hip joints. As I made the inventory, noting this involuntary activity, Pat was surprised to see what his body was doing. Up until that moment he had no idea that a large portion of his musculature had somehow slipped away from his voluntary control.

I then had him lie on his side with his knees drawn up and his head supported by a thick pillow. I palpated the long paravertebral muscles that rose vertically alongside the spine. They were highly contracted and quite hard to the touch, especially in the upper regions, which were sore, particularly on the right side. The spinal column was neither resilient nor straight; in the cervical and lumbar sections it was strongly curved, shortening the entire column. It was obvious that because of this chronic muscular tension Pat was less than his full height when he was standing. His entire frame was retracted, making him an inch or so shorter.

One aspect of the art of Functional Integration involves detecting any involuntary muscular activity that may be limiting the range and efficiency of intentional, voluntary movements. Once detected, it is possible to descry a specific pattern in these involuntary movements. This pattern is what I was looking for, because it is direct evidence of the state of the central nervous system in its sensorimotor activities. On the conscious level, Pat was incapable of voluntarily changing the contractions in his neck and lower back, so there was no point in addressing that level of his functions. But at the unconscious level of sensorimotor operations, if some change could be made, his condition might be improved. So I addressed myself to his sensorimotor functions, a realm where words could have no effect and where sensation of movement is the only language spoken.

When muscles are painfully contracted involuntarily, the last thing one should do is to attempt to pull the muscles and force them to release and lengthen; they will not do so. If one forces the muscle to lengthen, the immediate result is pain and increased involuntary contraction of the muscle. This is what had been done to Pat during the course of his earlier treatment, and it was this that had aggravated his condition.

Rather than trying to stretch the muscles forcibly alongside the spine, I moved the vertebrae laterally by lifting each vertebra an inch or so, then letting it settle back down. Pat felt movement in his otherwise painfully immobile vertebrae, but this sensing of movement involved no stretching whatsoever of the paravertebral muscles alongside the spine. It was comfortable movement, and almost immediately Pat involuntarily released a sigh of exhalation, which confirmed to me that the subject of my concern—the involuntary patterns of the sensorimotor system—were experiencing a comfortable relief. I lifted each vertebra from the pelvis up to the top of the rib vertebrae, then had him turn over onto the other side, where I repeated this procedure.

Finishing this, I asked Pat to lie on his stomach with his head turned to the right—the only direction in which he could comfortably face in the prone position. There I could clearly see the contracted curvature of the lumbar and cervical areas. I did not try to correct this curvature but, instead, did the reverse. I lightly encouraged the curvature of the lower back by softly pressing down on it. Pat sighed again, because this action of pressing down on the lower spine, increasing the curvature, had the effect of taking over the work of the paravertebral muscles, which themselves were involuntarily curving the lower spine. As soon as I began doing the work of these muscles for them, a curious thing automatically occurred: They began to relax, because they had no work to do; it was being done for them, so that their program of contraction became superfluous. Each time I pressed down, a certain degree of relaxation occurred in these muscles, so that at the end of the session I could feel that the muscles in the lower back and in the neck were slightly softer. Their involuntary program was being undermined.

This first session with Pat lasted some forty minutes, and

I did not see him until one week later. When he returned, he was no longer wearing the neck brace, he had ceased to take the pain pills, and he was astonished to report that almost all of the pain was gone for the first time in nine months. This is the typical physiological response that one looks for and usually finds in the practice of Functional Integration.

Although the acute pain had totally disappeared, soreness and stiffness were still there, yet to be reduced. During the next four sessions, I introduced him to other comfortable ways of moving, and the muscular tonus steadily dropped until there was only what he described as a "prickly" sensation in the rear, right side of his neck. But after the fifth session even this disappeared. Not definitively, however, because the next week he reported that he had felt a twinge of the prickly feeling return. It had occurred when he was at work—an important point to remember, since he was completely comfortable at home and during the weekend.

By the end of our ninth session Pat was beyond the point of worrying about pain; instead, he had phased into the positive stage, where his interest in athletics returned and he was playing baseball, tennis, and handling a sailboat by himself. The reeducation of the sensorimotor system of Pat was a success. He had, as it were, repossessed control of his musculature.

There was, however, a setback that, although only momentary, was highly significant. During the following summer's month-long vacation, he was as physically active and vital as he had ever been in his adult life. But at the end of three weeks an emergency caused him to return to his office in the city. He told me that as he was driving in, thinking of the difficulties he was going to have to solve in his agency, his neck began to pull again and by the next day was once again painful. This lasted only forty-eight hours, and by the time he returned for the last week of his vacation, his body was totally comfortable again.

The relation between Pat's stressful, high-tension business life and the involuntary tension of his muscles was obvious. His task now was to remain calm during the more anxiety-prone moments of his working day, and this he proceeded to do successfully by biofeedback training.

One further thing occurred that was fascinating. It had not been clear to me why the right rear section of his neck was the place of choice for his muscular distress, but during one of our last sessions, I was leading him through some subtle neck exercises, when he suddenly stopped and said, "My God! I just now remembered something that I haven't thought of for so long, I had completely forgotten it. When I was four, I had an attack of polio, and it centered in my neck, mainly in the section here on the right." The last mystery was solved. When one is under stress to the point of exhaustion, it is the weakest link that succumbs first.

Not only was Pat's response to these sessions typical, but also his distressed condition was typical. Such contractures of the neck are "normal" in our society, even though at times they appear totally mysterious. Sometimes the involuntary muscular activity is so inexplicable that the person feels he has been "possessed" by some strange force. One man whom I dealt with occasionally had such strong contractures in the upper regions of his body that his face became rigid; he told me that it felt like a giant hand had seized him, squeezing his face like a vise. A woman with whom I worked had frequent "attacks," when her face would become numb, the jaw rigid, and there were severe, throbbing headaches in her temples. In both cases, a few sessions of close attention to the specific pattern of their involuntary contracture delivered them from the "possession" and gave them back control of their muscles.

What, however, is not mysterious about these cases is that they involve severe retraction of the spine and that, in each and every case, these persons had been unhappily afflicted with severe and long-term stress. In the two cases of "possession" just mentioned there had been acute crises in their family lives.

When there is shortening of the spine, an individual shrinks. He literally becomes shorter in stature. Sometimes the shrinking is greater in the neck area; at other times it centers in the lower back. In either event, it is a common event in all urban civilization. Studies made in Great Britain and in Sweden indicate that at least half of the adult population suffers from some form of debility in the spine. The most common breakdowns occur in the lower back; less frequently they occur in the neck region. My own experience with somatic retraction indicates that in only 20 percent of such cases will there be greater contraction in the neck. Usually, the favored region is in the lumbar, so much so that what is called the lower-back syndrome is almost synonymous with being a businessman.

Bryan H. was a good example of this. A vigorous sixty-year-old retired businessman, Bryan began his retirement with a lower back so arched that, sitting, he could not lean over and touch his feet to put on his shoes—not simply because of the pain in his lumbar region but also because the contracted lumbar muscles prevented him from bending his back any further. This condition had endured for over ten years and was complicated by severe pains in his right hip joint. Bryan had some tightness in his neck, but it was minor compared with the swooping lordotic arch extending from his first lumbar vertebra to his pelvis.

Once the specific pattern of Bryan's involuntary contracture became clear, our sessions proceeded as follows: After the first session his lumbar muscles were relaxed and more extended, and the pain in the right hip joint became a mere soreness; after the second session, the lumbar was further lengthened, and all pain was gone from the hip joint; after the fourth session, Bryan could lean over and touch his foot for the first time in five years; after the fifth session, he could touch the floor alternately with each hand; after the sixth, he touched the floor with both hands —something he had not done for ten years—had a longer lower back and no pain or soreness of any kind. That was our last session together. Later, he phoned to say that he was again happily engrossed in the favorite obsession of his youth, hiking. Each week he joined a group of hikers for seven-mile treks under a full pack.

Anyone who has never experienced the muscular spasms that usually accompany the lower-back syndrome can have no idea of the devastating nature of the pain. The spasms will occur in the early morning to a man as he is bending forward over the basin to wash his face. They will occur when someone is coming out of the grocery store carrying a heavy bag. They typically occur to mothers, whose lower backs are taxed beyond tolerance as they lean over to pick up their babies. They happen to people who are weeding their gardens. Suddenly the lower back "freezes," "grabs," "catches," and the pain is so intense and so diffuse that the sufferer is completely immobile and cannot move for several days. The spasms are so overwhelming that, frequently, the person loses consciousness and needs to be hospitalized.

The extraordinary nature of the pain, whether in the lower back or in the neck, is so debilitating that all normal functions are wiped out. Appetite is gone, sexual potency is erased, there is no room for normal emotions or normal thinking. It is not simply the back that is in spasm; the entire being of the person is spastically frozen around a pain that is excruciating.

Obviously, this is not simply a muscular pain, and this is why those who have never experienced lumbar spasms are incapable of appreciating what it is like. To them the afflicted person appears to be exaggerating his pain, pretending to be helpless and weak rather than courageously struggling against it. What they do not understand is that the person has experienced not simply pain but a breakdown in vertical posture. The entire vertebral column is in jeopardy, because the curvature of the neck or lower back is so extreme that the weight of the head or—far worse—the weight of the entire trunk threatens to bend the curve so far that the neck or lumbar vertebrae would finally snap. What is experienced is the imminent possibility of breaking the neck or back and becoming paralyzed.

As I mentioned, the majority of adults in our society have retracted spines, usually in the lower back, and in each case, these adults have a lordotic arch in the lumbar region, caused by the unconscious and involuntary contraction of the extensor muscles lying to the right and left of the spine. People with lower-back syndrome are swaybacked, some slightly and others dramatically arched. This arch in the middle of their body means that if a heavy weight were placed on their head, the pressure would cause the back to bow out farther until it would literally break. If one were to take a long stick and place a significant weight on top of it, the stick would support that weight easily as long as its structure was in a straight line. But if one were to curve that stick, taking it away from the vertical line of its structure, and then place the same weight on top, the stick would bend and snap. This is precisely the threat that is experienced by the person having lumbar or cervical spasms: a threat to one's life.

When I first saw Richard W., he looked as if he was dying. A sixty-year-old man, his upper body was bent over almost horizontally, and he walked in a slow, lurching gait. He was pitiful. His eyes were pinched almost closed with the constant pain of ten years, his voice was hoarse, and his skin had collapsed into folds and wrinkles. Worse than that, he had about him the odor of despair, something one discovers in working closely with afflicted persons and that nurses in hospital wards are frequently aware of. The pains in his lower back had, over the ten-year period, been compounded with the appearance of sciatic pains, which coursed down his left leg. On the recommendation of an orthopedic surgeon he had submitted to an operation that involved surgical replacement of the ball of the left hip joint, using an aluminum ball for the head of the femur. This change in the structure of his hip did nothing to change the functioning of his hip or back. The same pains continued, and he hobbled into my office as a last resort.

Upon examining his body, I was not surprised to discover that his entire trunk was rigid with involuntary muscular contraction. The shoulder blades were frozen into immobility, the spinal column could not bend nor could the individual vertebrae rotate, the hip joints barely moved—particularly the left—and the interior muscles of the thighs were so tightly contracted that his legs could not open more than about six inches.

Having him lie down on his side, I proceeded to press on his vertebrae, making comfortable movements similar to what I described doing with Pat M. The result of this first session was that the sciatica entirely disappeared. The next week I worked with him while he was lying on his stomach. After twenty minutes of movements designed to release the extensor muscles on the sides of his lower spine, Richard was sound asleep. The relaxation of painful muscles after years of suffering was like a balm.

The relaxation meant one thing: that the involuntary contraction was being defeated and the muscles were now coming under Richard's voluntary control.

What I was introducing Richard to was movement—comfortable, normal movement of his muscles. During the next two sessions I gently induced him to begin rotating his torso. At first, he could turn farther to the right than to the left; then his rotational ability expanded and began to even out. By the end of the fourth session, he was standing erect, bending and moving his spine adequately and, best of all, he was without any pain in the lumbar region and the limp was imperceptible. Richard was beginning to look like a human being again. His skin no longer hung loosely, his eyes were twice as wide, his voice had a strong tone, and the forlorn smell of defeat was gone.

Now that he had attained confidence that he could regain control of his body, I asked Richard what specific goal he would like to set for the sessions ahead. He said that he had not been able, unaided, to put on his shoes for ten years, and he asked if I thought that was possible. I told him we would find out. I worked with Richard for five more sessions, at the end of which his back was limber enough that he could lean over and put on both shoes. Such an act may seem ludicrously simple, but for him it was a triumph. When he walked out the door saying goodbye, his eyes were lustrous, his posture vertical, and he had an immense watermelon smile that reminded me of Wallace Beery.

These cases are remarkable not because they are something exceptional but because they are normal. There are hundreds of similar cases. It is just as normal to have people respond the way Richard and Bryan and Pat did as it is for them to have been afflicted in the way they were. It is the predictable, expected norm of our society. But we cannot ignore the pathetic fact that the "normal" life that most humans lead is a life of unconscious self-destruction. If they were conscious of it, they would not do this to themselves, but as it is, they have no choice. They are hapless victims of a society in which a regular and insupportable burden of stress is consciously accepted as normal while, unconsciously, the central nervous system is brutalized to the point that it can no longer sustain the burden. Then the breakdown occurs; the person becomes conscious of it and is surprised that his body has somehow betrayed him.

The cases I have just described are instances of somatic retraction—retraction and shrinking not simply of the body but of the whole person. What the victim notices is that the bodily structure is painfully distorted. This structural distortion is also what the physicians and psychiatrists and psychotherapists notice, and they reply to the situation by attempting to do something with the bodily structure. This, however, is absolutely futile. The distortion of bodily *structure* is simply the last straw; it is the moment when the disintegration of the body's *functions* has endured so long and so intensely that the tissues can no longer support the constant functional stress.

Somatic retraction is a functional event. It is a sensorimotor response of the central nervous system. As such, it is beneath the level of words and beneath the usual range of daily consciousness. It takes place gradually and inexorably, muscles becoming more and more rigid and the sensory awareness becoming more and more muted. The atrophy of the proprioceptive and somesthetic senses is such an established event in the maturation of human beings that the unconsciously programmed destruction of the body takes place without the possessor of that body being either aware of it or capable of preventing it. What our culture accepts as the normal effects of aging are, to the contrary, the abnormal effects of our culture. Once, however, we understand the functional origins of this bodily distortion, we discover how this distortion is reversible.

This phenomenon of somatic retraction is a very special event. In characterizing it, I have used the words *cringing* and *shrinking.* This is precisely what the neuromuscular functions are doing in response to an intolerable stress. In somatic retraction, the functions draw the body inward, from the periphery toward the center, making it smaller. Not only is the spine shortened by muscular contraction around the lumbar and cervical vertebrae, but the arms and legs, shoulder joints and hip joints contract, flexing inward and narrowing the width of the body. It is the same cringing and shrinking response that occurs in all animals when they are frightened or stricken: They withdraw into themselves, becoming smaller, tighter, and less visible, as if, in order to protect themselves, they are attempting to disappear by pulling everything inward toward the center. In quadrupedal animals, this pulling inward of forepaws and hindlegs has the effect of dropping the animal down to the ground, the smallness and low visibility having survival value in face of the threat the animal perceives near it. Being small and motionless is a way of "playing dead." The living creature becomes tactically invisible by camouflaging itself with stillness. Since all animals recognize living being by the fact of movement, the predator is tricked by the lack of motion into believing there is no living body in the vicinity. In bipedal humans, the full and classic somatic retraction entails a flexion and adduction of the limbs and a bending of the spine at the two areas where there are no ribs to prevent it—the cervical and lumbar vertebrae, which are the most easily curved portions of the spine.

What I have been describing is not only a human reaction; it is, in the terms used in this book, a somatic reaction, which is to say that it is the way in which all living bodies react when their welfare and life are threatened. Somatic retraction is a functional response to a threat. As we shall see, it is not the only such response.

Commentary: The Function of Standing

Gravity is the cohesiveness of the cosmos. Without it, there would never have been an organized, rational, orbitally ordered universe—everything would have fallen asunder. Gravity is everywhere: in even the most remote corners of this immense universe it rules and orders the physical process, making things into efficient round orbits, into nice circles—it is a universal way of controlling the traffic of movement in the universe. Without gravity, movement would be random; with gravity, movement curves into circles.

There are laws of gravity, but gravity is not a law: It is an energy—and a perplexing energy, at that. It is an invisible energy, binding all bodies together. Its "attraction" between two or more bodies is created *by* those bodies: it is in the bodies themselves, and it is equally in the empty space between the bodies, filling the void of space with its binding presence.

Yet, it is an immaterial energy. Light energy is not immaterial: It zips through space in the form of photons or vibratory waves, both of which can be picked up and measured. Electromagnetic energy is equally measurable—its waves can be picked up by metals and crystals sensitive to its wave length. Chemical energy is measurable; more than that, it is visible through electron microscopes focused on molecular clusters. Heat is also a measurable form of energy, observably making its way from atom to atom, exciting them.

Gravity does not move through matter in waves, nor is

it composed of tiny specks of matterlike photons. Gravity is the ether of the universe—immaterial, omnipresent, and omnipotent. It rules the world and dictates its basic ground rules. Gravity is, if you will, the universe's nearest approximation to what theologians might call an immanent deity: namely, a God that is universal, ubiquitous, law-giving, and all powerful. I think it is quite impossible to conceive of the incredible nature of gravity without entertaining a quasitheological concept.

The somatic viewpoint seeks to understand life, first of all, by taking notice of the physical forces that have shaped the body of life. We know that the laws of the universe are the laws of life; so, to understand the one is to understand the other. To see life in terms of the three laws of thermodynamics is immediately to understand something about the process by which life organizes itself in ever more efficient ways. Far from demeaning the phenomenon of life and robbing it of its significance, such a viewpoint leads to the discovery that life, in its manifestation as *the soma, takes advantage of these universal laws and uses them for its advancement.* Living creatures have made a higher-order synthesis of the laws of thermodynamics, which govern matter, and have subsumed them within their process.

This awareness may very well arouse in us a further suspicion: *Is it possible that living beings take advantage of gravitational energy and use it for their advancement?* Is it possible that gravity does not dictate to the phenomenon of life and restrict it but, to the contrary, makes its extraordinary adventure possible?

From a purely human point of reference, gravity may seem to be negative: It makes things heavy, it creates weight and resistance, it is fatiguing. From the twig's-eye view, gravity may appear to be the enemy of life, the great limitation against which it has had to struggle every fatiguing step up the way. This, however, is not the case.

As we know, life began in the water, an environment whose buoyancy allowed the first soma to neutralize the downward pull of gravity and play with it. By being waterborne, the first soma was free: It had no weight and could go in any direction it wished. No atom can do that. No random molecular combination can do that. No planet can do that. No galaxy can do that. But the first somas could do that with no problem at all. Unlike other bodies in the universe, the body of life was, from the first, never weighed down by gravity; it used the gravitational cohesiveness of water molecules to bear up its three-dimensional shape, so that it would be free to expend its energies elsewhere.

Nothing in the history of life's evolution ever related to gravity other than as a neutral, supportive force. What makes this indisputable is that life did not stay in the water. If gravity was a danger, how could life have evolved into forms that gave up the buoyancy of water and moved onto the hard surface of earth? The answer is obvious: Somas evolved a way of being as buoyant on land as in the water. They did so by creating their own skeletal support (replacing the support of water) and a more complex neural system that could operate the soma somewhat more efficiently on land surface than in the sea.

Then, at some point in their land surface existence, somas became airborne—perhaps, at first, by sliding on the air like the flying squirrel who stretches out its arms to form a furry mantle and slides from one tree to another, using the cushion of air. From that point onward, it was a matter of gradually mutating the bones and flesh into lighter and more hollow structures. Then with the proper angles between bones and the proper muscles to move them, the arm-wing could be flapped, and the bird could go upward or downward just like a fish.

It is essential to understand that in the evolution from sea to land to air, nothing ever changed in the soma's relation to gravity. The soma, from the beginning to now, is buoyant and internally weightless; otherwise it would have fallen apart millions of years ago. Difficult as it may be to understand from our civilized human viewpoint, somas do not have "weight"; within themselves and to themselves, they have always known gravity as useful and ever supportive, just like the other forces in the universe.

Animals could not, of course, make use of gravity unless they had some means of recognizing it. They must have an organ capable of perceiving the vertical line of force always radiating upward from the earth's center. As we might expect, different animals have somewhat different organs of equilibrium by which they can tell immediately if their bodies are tilted off balance.

The organ of equilibrium in lower, invertebrate animals takes the form of a statocyst, a round organ whose inner walls are lined with sensory cells. At the bottom of this sensitive arena is a compact, heavy little ball called a statolith (literally, a "standing stone"). When the head of the animal tilts, the stone tilts away from the bottom of the statocyst and rolls against the sensory cells on one side, letting the animal know that it is no longer upright; if the tilt is to the other side, a different sensory message is sent to the central nervous system. In all somas, these organs of equilibrium evolved in relation to the rest of the soma's movements. When the organism senses that the statolith is off-center, this immediately triggers automatic countermovements to restore balance.

In some animals there is only one statocyst, and it is in the middle of the head. In others there are paired statocysts, stimulating left-side and right-side movements. If, by accident, one of the statocysts is out of order, an animal is likely to tilt and perhaps move about in a circle.

Most animals are chemically programmed to make their own statoliths. They secrete calcareous substances that form these gravitational stones. Other animals, notably the crustaceans, form their statocyst within a cranny of their shell, which has an external opening. With their claws they pick up a grain of sand and drop it into the opening—a straightforward way of supplying oneself with a gravitational stone. But since all crustaceans seasonally molt and lose their shells, they also seasonally lose their organ of equilibrium.

Knowing this, a zoologist named A. Kreidl performed an ingenious experiment with just-molted prawns. He placed them in filtered sea water that was devoid of sand or other particles; instead of sand, he supplied them with tiny iron particles, which the prawns promptly picked up and inserted in their newly forming statocysts. The iron particles worked quite well: Not only did they respond to the pull of gravity, but—unlike sand particles—they also responded to magnetic pull. What Kreidl did was to hold a strong magnet directly over the prawns, knowing that it would pull the iron statoliths out of position, drawing them straight upward toward the tops of the sensory walls. When the prawns experienced this change in the position of the gravitational stones, they "knew" that they were upside down. And what happened? When the magnet was held above the prawns, they immediately turned over on their backs and stayed there, feeling quite balanced and normal.

In the higher vertebrate somas the organs of equilibrium are much more sophisticated and do not require stones. In these animals, including the human, the balancing organ consists of sensory endings immersed in a fluid. When the fluid shifts back and forth during movement, it stimulates different sensory cells, informing the animal just how much it has moved from vertical center. These are enormously sensitive measuring devices, even in the lowliest animal. The slug worm—easily a candidate for the lowliest animal—can detect a change in its vertical balance when its body is tilted as little as one third of a degree.

By recognizing how this primeval sense of balance is automatically connected with a program of bodily movements, we realize how fundamental it is for somas to be upright. The slightest tilt from verticality and the entire mechanism goes into action to restore the body to balance. And if we recall a central feature of somas, their "stabilized instability," we quickly understand that gravity and the organs of equilibrium constitute a clear instance of how the soma is always restabilizing itself.

Because somas are always in motion, they are always losing balance. They therefore developed methods of restoring vertical balance, and these gravitational programs are instances of the general ability of all somas to stabilize and harmonize their functions so that they are maximally efficient.

This primitive relationship with gravity is basic to the bodily structure of the soma and the way it functions. It is by this upright function of standing that we can recognize the soma; nothing else in the universe is so stubborn about restoring itself to an upright position no matter how many times it loses balance.

Certain early human reflexes show us how primitive and powerful the standing function is. The human infant, its spine formed while in the fetal position and, at birth, devoid of any antigravity reflexes, soon begins to experiment with lifting the head. It is always remarkable to see a baby whose movements and muscles are scarcely developed suddenly lift its large head upward while it is lying on its stomach. This extension of the head upward is a search for verticality and equilibrium of the head over gravity. While in the fetal position the neonate had no curvature in the back of the neck or lower spine, but its drive to master gravity brings into action the extensor muscles in the back of the neck and, later, those in the back of the lower trunk. The infant is developing the normal curve of the cervical and lumbar regions, typical of the adult standing posture. By three or four months of age, when it is lying on its stomach, the infant explores all the ways it can arch its entire neck and back, including lifting its legs into the air. These are the child's first moves toward standing and walking.

Without the early development of the antigravity, extensor muscles, the baby would not learn to stand, nor, as we have learned, would other somatic functions develop, including the perceptual discriminations of normal intelligence. The same drive to lengthen and stand against gravity occurs in quadrupeds, all of whom have a profound distaste for lying on their back in the supine position. Automatically, they try to right themselves—just like the human infant—to lie in the prone position whereupon the extensor muscles in the legs and back contract to lift the body up above the ground.

"Standing up straight" is a sign of responsible adulthood, and, of course, the way in which all of us have learned to stand upright is by contracting the extensor muscles, particularly those in the neck and back. There is an optimal development of these antigravity, extensor muscles that guarantees comfort and efficiency in standing. Unfortunately, these muscles can, under certain circumstances, be provoked into contractions that take the spine past the point of optimal balance, creating hyperextension of the neck and/or lower back. Extreme curvature of the cervical and lumbar spine is the result of hyperextension, and this is what we have described as somatic retraction. This condition is directly related to intense and, usually, long-term stress.

Responsible human adulthood has meant to "stand on your own two feet," or "stand up like a man," both of which are thinly veiled commands to hyperextend the neck and lower back. The military drill posture of chin in, chest out, shoulders back, and knees locked backward is not thinly veiled at all. It is a command to distort the spine by deliberate hyperextension. The most common response to stress is to "stand up like a man," and we do it in the same unconscious, automatic manner that we first extended our backs during babyhood. It is as if, having taken our stance in the world by learning to stand straight (i.e., extended), we cannot help but respond to stress in the world by standing "straighter" (i.e., by hyperextension).

But "straighter" than straight is not straight at all; it is the curvature called lordosis, which plagues a large majority of the adult population.

The somatic retraction and shrinking caused by the superfluous effort of hyperextension is the characteristic way in which frightened people react. When faced with a threat, the normal human response is an energetic contraction of the extensor muscles, which gives one the internal feeling of being bolder and more defensively planted into the position one holds. In primitive human communities this reaction may last only so long as the threat is actually present—usually only briefly. In civilized human communities, however, the sustained threats and challenges to one's survival—real or imagined—create a sustained posture of fearful somatic contraction. Such a posture, maintained over a prolonged period, eventually results in painful spasms and general arthritic complaints.

But if somatic contraction is a fearful posture, pulling the body past the vertical line of "straightness," what are we to make of the inverse type of posture, whereby the standing body loses its "straightness" by collapsing forward in flexion? We must recognize that there are two ways of losing the optimum posture of uprightness. Somatic retraction is a very energetic distortion of the body, requiring sustained muscular extension, but somatic collapse is just the reverse distortion: It is the loss of energy and muscle tone and a folding forward into a flexed, fetal position. Somatic collapse is the posture that is found in human beings who are very old, weak, brain damaged, or schizophrenic. It is the posture of failure and falling. Therapists have observed that nonparanoid schizophrenics are typically slumped forward in flexion and have a fearful resistance to the head being tilted back in an extended position.

In sum, the optimal and efficient upright posture is a constant balancing between too little extension and too much—or too great a surrender to gravity and too great a defiance. The optimal balance—what Feldenkrais calls the potent posture—will display a tonicity of muscles that is equal between extensors and flexors. A balanced vertical stance means a balanced level of muscular tension. Viewed from the front, the spine will be absolutely vertical; viewed from the side, the spine will have compensatory curves that manage to keep the following points on the body in perfect vertical alignment: the meatus of the ear, the ball of the humerus, the ball of the trochanter, the midside of the knee, and the midside of the ankle bone. This is the optimal upright posture toward which the infant is developing, beginning with its first efforts to lift its head.

Just as surely as the spinal column is a central structural feature of the body, so is the action of standing a central functional feature. Before there was human culture and language, before there were human beings on this planet, there was the standing function, embodied in each and every soma.

To live is to move and to do so in a certain way. Somatic movement is not random; it has certain functional constants, and one of these is standing, with all the corresponding neural mechanisms that enable the soma to stand. All properly functioning somas seek to stand. Verticality and upwardness are the very signs of the healthy, efficiently operating soma.

Because standing is a general somatic function—and not

merely a bodily function—its presence indicates general efficiency in all aspects of our behavior: thinking, perception, emotions, judgment, and so on. Any disturbance in this general function necessarily means a general disturbance in all aspects of our behavior.

For example, there can be no psychological disturbance that is not accompanied by somatic distortion. Nor will the psychopathology disappear without the somatic distortion disappearing. Wilhelm Reich was the first psychoanalyst to point out the direct relationship between neurosis and the body. He observed that all neurotics have a disturbance of their sexual functions. This is undeniably true, just as it is equally true that *all* psychological states, whether healthy or pathological, are always the reflection of the sensorimotor activities going on in the bodily system. And when we see a disturbance in the standing function, we can be certain of finding general malfunctions within the whole human system.

Beneath the words and acculturation that are the focus of psychotherapy there is a subverbal realm of movement and sensation that is the primary determinant of health and efficient functioning. All of life stands upward against the vertical pull of gravity, the wondrous force that guided the body of life from its very first movements.

SOMATIC FIXATION

The structural center of the human body is the spinal column, just as the functional center of the body is the central nervous system. Structurally and functionally they are identical. All along the length of the spine the motor nerves exit from the front of the column, fanning out to the muscular tissues, causing them to contract when electrochemical impulses travel out through these motor nerves to the muscles they control. In the back of the spine, all along its length, the sensory nerves reach out to these same muscles, tendons, and joints, reporting back to the central nervous system their movements, angle of flexion, degree of contraction, and other information.

So, besides its structural purpose of supporting the weight of the upper body, the spinal column has the centralized functional purpose of relaying motor and sensory impulses between the sensorimotor cells in the periphery of the body and those in the central nervous system. The brain, which opens out like a flower at the top of the spinal column, reflects this same dominance of the sensorimotor functions. At the very top of the cerebral cortex are the sensorimotor tracts, stretching over the rounded surface of the brain above and between the ears. These tracts are separate from one another, the motor tract lying just to the front of center and the sensory tract just to the rear of center. From the top of the brain all the way down the spine we find the same rational plan: motor and sensory nerves at the center of the living body, with the former always to the front and the latter always to the back.

It is important to keep in mind that the brain has an orderly structure with a front, a back, and two sides. When we look at the head of a human being, we are simultaneously looking at the way the brain is structured: It is made to face forward. The optic nerves move forward to the two eyes, the olfactory nerves just underneath lead to the nose, and the hearing senses come out of the temporal lobes of the brain forming the ears which are also structured to face forward. These three senses are the teleceptors; they give the brain information of what is happening at a distance from the body.

These sense organs are thus fixed in a forward position facing the world outside. The eyes have a certain latitude of movement, as does the tongue, but they are nonetheless rooted in a fixed fashion in their assigned places in the front of the head. Even though the teleceptive senses are permanently fixed in one direction, the world surrounding us has 360 degrees of direction. If we wish to sense what is going on, we have no other option than to swivel the head around to the left or to the right, pointing the face whichever way we want to point the teleceptors. This means that the structural and functional center of our body—the spinal column—must be capable of rotating the head in whatever direction we need to face.

In primitive societies, whether living in forests or on the open plains, survival clearly depends on the ability to be aware, through one's teleceptors, of what is happening on all sides of us. The ability to turn and face in any direction is a survival function not simply of human beings but of all living creatures from amoebas to mammals. Only circular-structured animals, such as sea anemones and starfish, have a face and body that is fixed and immobile; their mode of survival is, like plants, much simpler, for they prefer clinging to one spot.

So, for compelling reasons that are biologically obvious, human beings must have the ability to rotate the head in any direction they need. It is the spinal column that makes this survival function possible. Just under the skull and supporting it are seven cervical vertebrae, and these in turn are stacked on top of seventeen thoracic and lumbar vertebrae, all of which have the power of independent movement and rotation. Taken together, these twenty-four vertebrae give the human torso and head such an enormous range of rotational movement that it would seem inconceivable that this highly flexible structure could ever fail to be able to turn. Yet it is possible, not because of something that goes wrong with the structure of the spine but because of something that is wrong with its functioning, namely, the working of the central nervous system. When this inconceivable event happens, the human being is in danger and his survival chances are suddenly decreased.

This was the situation of a man who hobbled into my office one March morning. He was a fifty-five-year-old pharmacist named Larry F. Larry's trunk was bent at a 20-degree angle, and he walked in a ducklike manner, the trunk bobbing alternately to the left and to the right. He told me that the medical diagnosis was that he had a displaced fifth lumbar vertebra with sciatica, the pains being felt in the left hip joint. The right hip joint was also extremely sore. Standard medical treatment had not relieved the problem, nor had visits to a chiropractor. As a pharmacist, he was on his feet all day and had to be able to stand comfortably. As it was, however, he was too painfully crippled to continue in his occupation.

I had him lie down so that I could examine the way in which his body moved. Larry was a short, stocky man with a powerful barrel chest. While he was lying on his right side, I pushed slightly on the right section of his pelvis to see how easily it could tilt forward. It did not move. I pulled backward, and there was no movement in this direction either. Then moving up to his arms, I put my hand behind the right shoulder blade and, again, pressed it forward. It, too, refused to move. Then I took his head in both hands to see how much the neck could turn. Once again, there was no movement. I pressed on his ribs, bones that are quite soft and pliable if the intercostal muscles are relaxed. It was like pressing on a steel cage; his ribs were solidly immobile. Larry's entire trunk, from pelvis to head, was like a single block of cement. It was most extraordinary. I felt as if I were pressing upon some nonliving substance, a statue that looked like a man but was made of marble.

I then turned my attention to his legs. I slowly lifted the

right leg and rotated it a few degrees. It turned, but somewhat jerkily and painfully. At least there was movement. I discovered that the left leg also allowed movement. When I had finished the examination of his movement functions, I could see that there was no movement of his body from the pelvis upward; only the legs moved from the hip joints downward.

So the functional picture that emerged was this: Over a certain number of years, Larry had progressively moved his torso less and less, even ceasing to move the shoulder blades when he reached forward with his hands to fill prescriptions. But how was it possible to move at all, if the trunk was a monolithic, undifferentiated block? The answer was obvious: by moving the hip joints. When Larry reached forward, he did so by tilting his entire trunk forward from the hips. When he turned to the left or right, he did so by moving only the hip joints and ankles. When he walked, he activated only the hip joints. In sum, the entire burden of moving the heavy upper trunk fell directly upon the hip joints, whose muscles were so overworked that they were in chronic pain. He did not have sciatica; it was not a nerve pain he felt but the excruciating burning feeling of muscles whose fibers have been so continually abused that, as in a recruit forced to do a thirty-mile march under full pack, the muscles were exquisitely sore.

Given this functional situation, what could one do to reverse such a strange combination of upper-body immobility and lower-body abuse? It seemed obvious that the hip joints needed to be relieved of their constant overwork and that the only manner of achieving this was to reawaken movement in the torso. There was nothing structurally wrong with his hip joints, but there was everything functionally wrong with his entire spinal column: It could not rotate. It was as if, over the years, Larry had forgotten how to move his vertebrae—a kind of somatic amnesia.

Muscles that do not move are muscles that are not sensed. There must be movement in order to stimulate the sense endings within the muscle and in the joints. This is to say that Larry's "amnesia" was not only that he had forgotten how to move the spinal and upper trunk muscles; he had also forgotten what these muscles felt like. The sensory awareness he had of his trunk was devoid of any feeling of having seventeen different vertebrae or of having individual ribs or of having shoulders that are separate from the rib cage. His proprioceptive abilities of self-sensing were inactive. Within his trunk he felt almost nothing. Indeed, the main thing he felt in his body was the constant pain in his hip joints.

Looked at in objective physiological terms, Larry's motor system was largely inactive; but a purely objective, physiological viewpoint misses the full picture, namely, that this muscular stillness means a sensory stillness. Larry's awareness was receiving no sensory feedback from his muscles. From the internal point of view of his consciousness, he no longer had a trunk. It had not simply ceased to move; for him, it had ceased to exist.

So, during this first session I began "reminding" him of the existence of his trunk. While he was on his side, I began to press around the borders of his shoulder blade, touching the muscles of the scapula that radiate out to other sections of the trunk. By thus working my way around the entire rim of the scapula, I myself was lightly moving

Larry's muscles, thereby activating the sensory cells. Internally, from Larry's point of view, I was sketching out a neural picture of his shoulder blade, a picture he had somehow forgotten. In a nonverbal manner I was "showing" him his own shoulder blade.

By pressing on the muscles and creating new sensory information, a very special process begins to take place. The sensory stimulation of those particular muscles goes directly to the sensory tract in the cerebral cortex, which is lying alongside the motor tract. This stimulation of the sensory endings around the shoulder blade diffuses into the motor neurons controlling the muscles in exactly the same area I was touching. By sketching a neural picture of his scapula, I was simultaneously stimulating the motor neurons into activity.

Once the neural picture was sketched for him, I pressed on the medial edge of the scapula, and a wonderful thing happened: It moved. Not much, but it moved. Then I pressed in the opposite direction on the lateral edge of the shoulder blade, and it moved back slightly. Profiting from this new mobility, I pushed on the lower, medial edge of the blade, moving it slightly upward and outward. Then, changing my position, I pressed on the upper, lateral edge of the bone, and succeeded in moving it downward and inward.

Following this procedure until I had worked my way completely around the scapula, I was able to bring movement into the right shoulder blade in all directions. I then had him turn over, and I repeated the same operation on his left shoulder with the same results. I was *teaching* Larry to move his shoulders again by teaching him that he had two shoulder blades. The lesson he was learning was a purely nonverbal lesson given to his sensorimotor system. Before he could *move* his shoulders, he had to have the sensory awareness of *having* shoulders. By the time the first session had ended, Larry had begun to move his shoulders.

During the second session I gave the same sensory lesson to his ribs and lower back, with the result that the vertebrae began to move and rotate. The movement of the torso was sluggish, but it moved—and it moved because Larry himself was moving it. He was regaining the sensory awareness and the movement he had lost. He had become aware of having not simply a torso but a torso that was differentiated into many parts—two scapulae, two clavicles, and more vertebrae than he ever remembered having.

When he returned for the third session, he brought good news: He was standing erect, with almost no limp, and all pain in the hip joints had disappeared. To say that he was pleased would be an understatement. During that hour we worked to widen the range of his spinal rotation, so that, from the facing position, he could turn 80 degrees to the left and 80 degrees to the right, that is, he could turn his trunk at almost a right angle to his pelvis, something that not even all athletes can do.

He departed in high spirits and great expectations. Too great, in fact. I neglected to warn him that the results of Functional Integration frequently seem so effortlessly magical that my clients often need to guard against premature aspirations of athletic grandeur. When he returned for the fourth session, he was limping again and the left hip joint was sore. I asked him what had happened. Sheepishly he confessed that he had celebrated the end of his hip joint pain by—of all things—going out with friends for a round of golf. He took a mighty swing at the ball with his driver, twisting his just-awakened torso into a full rotation as he did his follow-through. But his torso was hardly prepared for such enthusiasm, nor was his hip joint, and his sensory cells loudly informed him that he had made a mistake.

The hip joint was not, however, painful—only sore, and the soreness was gone within forty-eight hours. We had two more lessons, and at the end of the sixth session Larry was comfortable and supple, fully capable of playing golf again. Not only had the pain and immobility disappeared, but in movement and spirit he said that he felt as if twenty-five years had disappeared, leaving him feeling as if he was age thirty again.

From a medical standpoint, Larry could not be helped; he was an "incurable." And the fact that he could be taken from a crippled condition to a semiathletic one in six hour-long sessions is a source of amazement to anyone who is not acquainted with Functional Integration. But once such happenings are seen over and over again, the amazement fades, and another question arises about another surprising fact. Larry's entire spine had been frozen into immobility, incapable of rotating: How is it possible for a human being to "forget how to turn"?

In our discussion of somatic retraction, it was shown that a living body will shrink inward from periphery to center when it is forced to function in a condition of threat, fear, or heavy challenge, that is, under a condition of intense or sustained stress. The outward source of the stress is the effective cause of the functional response of bodily retraction. In the case of Larry, the somatic distortion that occurred was not one of spinal retraction but rather one of spinal fixation. There was no significant presence of contraction in the extensor muscles of the cervical and lumbar vertebrae. The fixing of the spine in one direction, always facing forward, is a distinctly different event, having to do with the movement of the body in a different plane. In retraction, the human's vertical plane of stature is reduced and shortened downward; in fixation, the human's horizontal plane of movement around the vertical spine is reduced and limited laterally in its rotation.

I have discovered that when a functional distortion occurs in a different spatial plane, it represents a different response to a different situation. Although I frequently work with clients whose bodies show both somatic retraction and somatic fixation, the two conditions are categorically distinct.

If Larry had asked me why it was that he had somehow become stuck in one position, incapable of rotating his spine, I would perhaps have asked him to compare his day-to-day movements, habits, and thoughts with those that he had had twenty-five years ago, when he was thirty. I would have asked him to compare the variety of what he did then with the variety of what he does now. I would have asked him whether he thought that, during the past twenty-five years, his life had taken on greater richness and newer directions or had it become narrower and ever more specialized. I would have asked him if the aspirations and challenges and hopes and fears that he had now were anything as complex and numerous as when he was thirty.

One of the myths of aging is that we cannot do all the things that we once could do. But the actual fact about aging is that we cease to do all the things that we once did. As our search for a vocation settles into a fixed "job," as our search for a mate settles into marriage, as our many expectations settle into a finite number of fulfillments, as our aspirations settle into steady certitudes, and as our broad range of potential movements settles into a narrow band of habitual movements, we will inevitably find ourselves looking in fewer directions and moving in fewer directions. As the possibilities of our life are sorted through, discarded, and finally edited down to a daily routine of actualities, our living functions become limited and specialized.

Larry's life was invariable, just as are the lives of many adults. The accepted personal goal of "adulthood" is, it seems, to settle down and obtain security, to obtain a fixed pattern of life that allows us to escape from the insecurity of freedom and the incertitude of new aspirations. To the degree that individual human beings are seduced into the accepted belief that personal fulfillment means a settled, secure, and circumscribed mode of life, so, to that degree, do the functions of one's living body adapt, becoming simpler, more straightforward, and rigid.

Larry had ceased to look around. He no longer felt that he needed to look around. After all, what more is life than to cease looking around and to settle down? This is exactly how Larry functioned. His daily life had become less and less varied and more and more specialized. In the same way that twenty-four vertebrae had ceased to be sensed and moved, becoming, as it were, fused into a single, undifferentiated block, so had the awareness and potential actions of Larry become fused into a unidirectional life.

And for this same reason, once the effects of his unthinking, unquestioned acculturation were undermined by my "lessons" at the nonverbal and, thus, subcultural level of his sensorimotor awakening, Larry became more aspirational and adventurous. More was now possible for him, and he could look around more and aspire to more. I am suggesting that living human beings, when they are understood somatically in terms of their living, moving functions, reveal themselves "psychologically" exactly to the same degree that they reveal themselves "physiologically." "Mind" and "body" are revealed simultaneously by the same living individual, the living human soma. And the somatic repertoire of this individual can grow and become richer, or it can diminish and become poorer. There is a parable about this, recorded by Saint Matthew, and it ends with the following judgment: "For unto every one that hath shall be given, and he shall have abundance: but from him that hath not shall be taken away even that which he hath. And cast ye the unprofitable servant into the outer darkness: there shall be weeping and gnashing of teeth." And there also shall be no rotation of the spinal column.

Although it occurs in females, somatic fixation is typically a male phenomenon. It is a psychophysiological state that is immediately associated with a male who is steady, reliable, and utterly committed to a single role. Most commonly, such a male shows his personal life to be indistinguishable from his professional-vocational life. He has totally habituated his living behavior to that role with a minimal intrusion of personal difference or unexpectedness. From a certain point of view, to be somatically fixed, always facing resolutely in one direction, is a virtue: The invariable man is a dependable man. He can be counted on to continue doing the same things and to do them in the same direction. One suspects that bank directors think of this kind of man as an ideal bank officer.

In American culture somatic fixation is more common in small towns and rural communities, where fixed and steady roles are encouraged and rewarded. As such, there is something "old-fashioned" about human beings who are somatically fixed. It is a type of rigid role-playing that is more typical of traditionalized urban societies, whether European or Asian. In Europe, for example, it is a form of somatic behavior more encouraged by the Teutonic cultures than by the Latin ones; the incidence of "stiff-backed" and "stiff-necked" people is visibly higher in these cultures. Most notably it is a phenomenon associated with royalty and aristocracy in all cultures. The French, Italian, or Spanish aristocrat, born and bred to identify proudly with his inherited role, is trained into somatic fixation and has a bearing that is in sharp contrast to that of the loose-spined commoners of these same cultures. It is here, among the aristocracy, that one finds women who are on an equal footing with men in terms of somatic fixation. The stiff, straight-ahead, "regal" bearing of an aristocratic French matriarch in her sixties suffers not at all in comparison with that of a male Prussian Junker.

When I have worked with persons whose spines are rigidly nonrotational, I always notice that they are unaware of this rigidity. As in all cases of somatic distortion, the sensorimotor atrophy has taken place without their knowing it. I once asked a banker in his fifties to rotate his pelvis to the left. I watched him, waiting for him to move, and then, thinking he had not heard me, said, "Go ahead and rotate to the left." He said, "I just did." So I said, "Try rotating your pelvis to the right." I waited. There was not the least movement. I asked, "Have you moved?" and he said, "Yes." In his own awareness, he believed he had moved, because he intended to, but when the sensorimotor functions are atrophied, intentions count for nothing: The man is effectively paralyzed.

In orthopedic medicine, physicians occasionally see an unusual disease that they call ankylosing spondylitis—"spondylitis" referring to a painful rheumatoid arthritis of the spine and "ankylosis" referring to the gradual fusion of the spine into solid bone. It is a frightening disease and an inexplicable one; no one has discovered any cause of it. The disease simply occurs, perhaps from genetic predisposition. The ailment begins in the sacroiliac joints in the back of the pelvis and gradually moves up the spine, causing pain. The individual can still flex and extend the spine, but it is almost impossible to rotate it. As the spine becomes progressively more immobile, cartilage and bone destruction occurs and ankylosing begins—namely, the vertebrae begin to fuse, creating what is called a poker spine. Eventually, calcification builds up until the entire vertebral column is encased in a calcium shell and the spine is totally immobile. The disease is not lethal. The patient continues to live and can walk and perform limited movements.

From a somatic viewpoint, all diseases without any known cause are intriguing, for they point to factors about which physiological medicine knows almost nothing. Perhaps the most fascinating aspect of ankylosing spondylitis is that in 90 percent of cases the victim is a male within the age range of twenty to forty—a statistic that strongly suggests that, as the result of genetic and/or cultural factors, the unyieldingness and unturningness of somatic fixation are functionally identified with the male role. If this is the case, it shows us that the ancient and traditional ideal of the resolute, irrefragable, absolutely reliable adult male is an ideal that can be achieved only by a steady attrition of the male's awareness and motor capacities. Somatic amnesia is the precondition for somatic fixation.

We have, then, two forms of somatic spatial distortion: (1) somatic retraction, which in human beings is a retrenchment of the vertical line in which we stand; and (2) somatic fixation, which is a frontal rigidity. These two distortions of the spatiality of the living body are distinguished from one another both in the ways they are formed and in the ways they finally manifest themselves.

Commentary: The Function of Facing

Some of the characteristics of life are so commonplace that we tend to overlook them. That is the mark of a primordial characteristic: It is something so universal that it hovers just below the threshold of our consciousness. The fact that all somas stand upright in balance with gravity is one such characteristic. Another common and universal trait of somas is their face.

Perhaps, since somas are structures that *function,* it would be more correct to say that *the function of facing is a basic characteristic of life.* It is odd that we should notice that living things have faces without realizing that the part of the body called the face is made for facing the world.

The function of facing is more important than the face itself, if we are to believe one of the simplest of all living creatures, the amoeba. Amoebas do not have much of a fixed structure at all. There is a membrane and the cytoplasm within it but there is no face, no front, nor is there a back. But the amoeba faces the world just the same. When it wants something, it moves toward it by extending and planting little hands and fingers called pseudopods; then, once this advanced beachhold has been established, the amoeba begins pouring its cytoplasmic self forward into the new space it has created. It could just as well have gone in any other direction, because it is not burdened with a bodily structure that has a front and a rear—a head and a tail. But it can do without the somatic structure, just as long as it has the somatic function. It heads into the world exactly like any other living being.

It is the nature of the soma to "head into the world," and this is so for a simple reason: Somas are always moving. When the soma moves, it faces the world and heads into it—or, if the going is rough, it may back away from the world and flee.

In so simple a creature as an amoeba, the decision to take the shape of a head and tail has not yet been made. The function is there, but the structure is absent. The amoeba is not alone in lacking a head and tail. The entire plant world attempts to avoid it, as do certain round or radial animals, such as sponges, jellyfish, and starfish. Even within their own phylum of Protozoa, which numbers in excess of a quarter of a million species, amoebas are an exception to the rule that somas have a head–tail structure. The other classes of one-celled animals tend to show an elementary head structure that leads movement and a tail structure that follows behind.

It is movement that creates the head–tail structure. It is

the function that dictates the structure. Biologists are familiar with this feature of life. When they see a special bodily structure, their first question is, What is its function? What is it made for? Any bodily structure that exists has evolved and survived because it serves some general function of helping the animal live and spread its progeny. So when we observe any general feature of anatomy, our own initial reaction should be, What is its function? If we see a universal tendency among somas to have heads and tails, then we know that this signals a universal and primordial function in somas: movement forward.

By the same token, if we see simple somas, such as plants, sponges, and starfish, without a clear head–tail structure, then we know that they have little concern with moving forward. Rather, they are planted in one place or they are drifting, willy-nilly, with the currents of water.

Plants do not need independent movement to survive; they do very well without it. Rather than moving about, looking for nutrition, plants station themselves in the midst of an adequate nutritional terrain. To say that they "station themselves" is to point out that plants, like all other somas, have the primordial function of standing upright in balance with gravity: They shoot their roots downward and their bodies upward.

The ability to move forward is not totally absent in plants; plants need sun and carbon dioxide, and they will reach toward these necessities. For example, vines will go through ingenious contortions to climb up to a patch of light. Leaves and flowers not only open and close to light, but they will turn and follow the light with their "faces" as the sun courses from east to west.

It was one of Charles Darwin's great delights to show

biologists that the dividing line between plants and animals is not a very sharp one. Sponges illustrate this ambiguity. Until two hundred years ago biologists were certain that sponges were plants. After all, they rooted themselves to stationary objects and looked like plants. But in 1766 John Ellis discovered that sponges vigorously eject currents of water through their tubes. Later it was found that sponges lacked an ingredient native to all plants, cellulose. Moreover, both a rudimentary muscle system and a rudimentary nervous system have been detected. So sponges are animals, but they are such curious animals and so plantlike that they are ambiguously classified as Parazoa—neither a multicelled animal nor a colony of single-celled Protozoa but a curious admixture. Darwin saw that the same functions were present in plants, even though muted. In the greenhouses of his Down estate he was elated to prove that, contrary to the belief of biologists, plants such as the Venus's-flytrap have a gastric system for digesting their catch!

Somas either move toward something or away from something, and the bodies of animal somas reflect this line of movement: *They elongate.* If a soma is stationary, its most efficient form is circular, but if it moves, its form becomes more streamlined. This streamlining means not only a change in its outer shape but a change in its inner shape as well. Certain organs move toward the "front" and are balanced around a central line, the long neural cord that will later develop into a spinal cord. The preferred shape of all advanced somas is an elongated body. There is a head at the front end, housing the sensory apparatus, and this trails back through the neural cord to the tail. This shape fits its function, which is to go forward.

To reach an understanding of life, it is crucial to realize that, even at its simplest levels, *life's tendency is to move forward.* Both the elemental structure and the function of life's body testifies to the fact that the movement of life is neither relative nor indifferent: Life intends to move forward.

All somas move forward *toward* something. This lets us know that, even at the most elementary level, living things have some kind of guidance system. That is why, in the soma's elongated body, the sense organs are in the head and are exposed at the face: The soma must sense where it is going in order to correct its course. Thus something as tiny and simple as a one-celled paramecium is a classically self-guiding cybernetic system.

There is yet one more remarkable consequence of the soma's tendency to move forward: It possesses a sensorimotor system. Even though there may be no nerve cells, the sense function is operative. Even though there may be no muscle fibers, the motor function of contraction is operative. It appears that all somatic functions precede somatic structure. Certain physical laws that were incorporated into the higher-order synthesis of somas dictate the kind of structural possibilities that will evolve. The same general somatic function may have a thousand different structural expressions. A snake, a bird, a frog, and a monkey are all made to move forward, yet their bodily structure, their skeleton and joints, their musculature, the position of their sense organs, and the arrangement of their central nervous system are quite diverse.

Let me emphasize how startling it is that all of these crucial somatic traits—elongation, head-tail structure, intentionality, and a sensorimotor guidance system—come from a single, primordial function, that of facing and moving forward. This is all the more astonishing when we realize that this function is imposed upon the soma by the physical universe. Any body in the physical world must have three spatial dimensions: length, depth, and width. I have already described the first dimension of space imposed on the soma: the uprising extension of limbs and body above gravity. This created the function of standing upright. The second spatial dimension is that of depth, which constitutes the first of two horizontal planes. This second spatial dimension guarantees that somas will have a cranial–caudal bodily structure. This is a most useful structure, not only because it is streamlined but also because, like an arrow, *it points*—it is already mobilized in one direction.

From a purely structural point of view, the soma need not be pointed any more than it need be round or square. But from a functional point of view, such a pointed structure is obvious.The soma is an energy system made possible through a higher-order synthesis of elements. We have already noticed how efficient an antientropic energy system it is. It has more energy than it needs simply to exist as a body. Since the soma floats on gravity through some form of buoyancy, this surplus energy is available for movement along the horizontal plane.

But along which horizontal plane shall the soma's excess energy be directed? The answer to this is obvious, since we know that the laws of thermodynamics are responded to with utter efficiency in the operations of the soma. Inasmuch as movement in any direction would, as with the amoeba, demand reorganizing the entire bodily structure for each movement, then it is better to specialize along one line, with the body always premobilized for a forward movement.

Also, every living being larger than a single cell has a face. From elementary biology to advanced psychology the same somatic law prevails: All living creatures eat their way through the world; their appetite guides their open maws toward the nutritional energy they require.

The face is the most needful part of a soma and its most sensitive part. To other somas the face is the most expressive part of the soma. Every creature watches the face of the other in order to know what he is intending. Animals watch the mouth, the show of teeth, the flesh around the eyes, the position of the ears—all of these tell the animal what the other is up to.

In his epochal *The Expression of the Emotions in Man and Animals,* Charles Darwin was the first to describe the typical expressive movements of animals, indicating their intentions of attacking or fleeing. The angry dog who is about to attack brings his ears forward, raises his hind quarters, and opens his mouth, exposing the canine teeth. The frightened or docile dog lays his ears back, smooths his back downward, and pulls back the corners of his lips.

Konrad Lorenz and his associates have created detailed charts in which fight and flight behavior are specifically indicated in large numbers of different animals. These ethological studies do not, fortunately, end with subhuman animals but include us, the human species. In this respect, ethology has been one of the great teachers of the somatic point of view, seeing human behavior as already prefigured in earlier somatic behavior. We might not otherwise realize, for instance, that when a human being sneers, he is baring his canine teeth just like a canine or feline ready to attack.

We have faces because we are made to move forward. That is not a psychological fact; it is a somatic fact. *All animals look at what they want.* If an animal did not face what it wanted, did not look at what it wanted, and did not move toward what it wanted, we would know without doubt that it was either sick or frightened. This is important to know in human psychology: Does a person face directly into the world? Are the face and head straight and erect? Does he look directly at other people, or does he slightly avert his eyes? These questions are appropriate at any organic level, from mice to men.

The somatic understanding seeks to take fuller account of the history of life and its many layers. We learn about life *from* life, from its diversity and its many-textured history. The French philosopher Maurice Merleau-Ponty talks about life's history in geological terms. He speaks of life's "sedimentations," one layer gradually covering another layer, like the expanding growing circles of a tree trunk or the gradual layering-out of the mineral sediments of the earth.

Life is like the historical structure of an onion, one layer resting on and enveloping the preceding layer. And understanding life without gross distortion means to peel this onion, layer by layer. In the onion, as in the evolutionary tree of life, each layer reveals underneath it a lower layer that is similar but a bit smaller and simpler. Each layer shows a change, but not that much of a change. It is only by keeping track of these incremental decreases in the scope of the onion peel that we begin to see the obvious. And how obvious these truths are is confirmed by how consistently they narrow their path directly back to the centrum. The basic somatic patterns—or, if you will, the patterns of life—are those that have consistently prevailed throughout all somas, from the simplest and earliest to the most complex and recent. To know these patterns is to know that living things have certain simple and basic ways of functioning.

Standing is one of these elementary patterns. *Facing* is another. They are living functions that are so familiar and obvious that we can confirm their fundamental importance simply by noticing that every other living creature also stands and faces.

In human beings, however, the function of facing has evolved an additional feature: the ability to focus one's awareness in any direction one wishes. In all acts of conscious attention we mobilize the whole of our sensorimotor system along the line of a trajectory, pointing at something in the external world or, when the occasion invites it, pointing at something within our internal world. We can mobilize consciousness in only one direction at a time for the same reason that we can only face in one direction at a time: A single, individual soma whose system is wholly mobilized to face in one direction has nothing left in its system to face elsewhere. To face in a new direction requires reorganizing and remobilizing the entire system as a unit.

Whereas nonhuman somas inherit a phylogenetic program for the ways in which they shall face, human beings have freed themselves from such phylogenetic programs. Through our use of language we have replaced these programs of biological direction with educational programs of cultural direction. Somatic educators have urged us to take advantage of this freedom by focusing our awareness inward upon certain internal processes of our body. This ability to mobilize the sensorimotor system, isolating one particular movement of our body, makes it possible to integrate that newly discovered movement into the general process of our central nervous system, making us more efficient and adaptable.

By saying that the functions of standing and facing are primordial, it makes them sound very old and remote—which they are not. No matter how long ago a function first appeared, so long as it survives, it will always be new and fresh. The functions of life cannot grow old.

The original body of life still lives.

SOMATIC LATERALIZATION

"What you don't know can't hurt you" is a saying that is as false as it is familiar. Ignorance of the internal process of our bodies can destroy us, and it does so regularly. Far better the dictum "Know thyself," inscribed on the temple at Delphi.

Usually it is the external world that absorbs our attention. The persistent pressures and challenges of our social and physical environment can keep us so distracted from ourselves that internal strains and imbalances can build up slowly and imperceptibly. Often a client with a painfully distorted body will look up at me and ask, "How could a thing like this happen to me?" Of course, the answer is that the disability that eventually thrusts itself painfully into his awareness had been happening all the time, slowly, just beneath the threshold of his consciousness. If, during the course of this gradual buildup, he had turned his attention inward, he might have noticed what was happening. But adults rarely make use of their faculties of self-sensing.

The turning of one's attention inward is a powerful agent for change. Focusing one's attention is not simply a psychological act of passive perception; rather, it is a positive, physiological act. To gaze outward at a tree will not affect the tree, but to gaze inward at oneself is a radically different act that cannot fail to affect oneself.

Something remarkable happens when we direct our attention inward. If a person stops for a moment and focuses his awareness on his left ear, the ear becomes highlighted. Only a second earlier, it was submerged in an undifferentiated obscurity, but now it is limned by a neural spotlight that causes it to stand out like a prominent figure against the obscure background of the rest of one's body. Focusing awareness on one portion of the body is a most special sensorimotor action, because it not only mobilizes the sensorimotor system in one direction but it simultaneously inhibits its focus in all other directions. This is to say that it is an action involving the entirety of the sensorimotor system and, thus, the entirety of one's body.

Just as we can face in only one direction at a time, so also can we focus our awareness in only one direction at a time. What we turn our consciousness toward may be either immensely complex or infinitely simple, but it is always toward one thing only. It is from this unidirectional focus, excluding all other directions, that the mobilizing power of directed awareness is gained. It is sufficient to recall the procedure of drawing a "neural picture" of Larry's shoulder, an action that allowed him not only to become aware of his shoulder blade but to begin moving it.

Most probably, you and I were not aware of which sock or shoe we put on first this morning. It is quite conceivable that someone could live his whole life without ever noticing which leg he always puts into his trousers first. Few persons notice which leg they habitually stand on, nor are they aware of which arm is always on top when their arms are crossed, which leg is on top when their legs are crossed, or which thumb is on top when their fingers are interlaced. Yet, for almost everyone there is a consistent, habitual way in which we do these things, and it is directly linked to the fact of lateral dominance—that is, whether we are right-handed or left-handed.

Usually when a right-handed person interlaces his hands, the right thumb will be on top of the left thumb. Usually, this same right-handed person will insert his right leg into his trousers first; a left-hander will do the opposite. Usually, a right-handed person will automatically put more of his weight on the left leg, leaving the right leg free. This is because, for him, the right leg—and all of his right side—is more "intelligent" than the left. If he wishes to put a toe into the swimming pool to see how cold the water is, he will put in the right foot while standing on the left. If he kicks a ball, he will do so with his "smart" and better controlled right foot, pushing off from the left foot. I say usually. Sometimes this is not the case, and when it is not, there may be trouble.

When I first see a client, I always ask him to stand still with his eyes closed while I study his vertical posture from the front. When someone is standing still, there will generally be a straight, vertical line coming down from the nose and chin cleft through the center of the breastbone, the navel, and the center of the pubis. Likewise, the two shoulders are expected to be on an even, horizontal line and also the two sides of the pelvis. This, however, is not always the case.

Often when I look at a person who is standing facing me, I will see that the right shoulder is slightly lower than the left. Frequently this person's head will be tilted a little to the right. Also, if I look very closely, I may notice that his right hip joint is higher than the left, making the right hip joint nearer to the right shoulder than the left hip joint is to the left shoulder. If I were using a fluoroscope, I would see a number of other things occurring within this person's body: The ribs on the right side would be more compressed than the ribs on the left side, and the entire spine would be held in a scoliotic curve. Moreover, if I asked him which leg seemed longer, he would most likely say it was the left and that he has always been told by tailors that his right leg was shorter than the left. If I were to place my hand on his back and compare the degree of hardness between the paravertebral muscles on the right side with those on the left side of the spinal column, I would find that the muscles were clearly tighter on one side than on the other. And when one adds up all these features, in light of the fact that a normally formed skeleton will always be in symmetrical balance unless the muscles attached to it are distorting its balance, the following picture emerges: The habitual—and normally unconscious—pattern of this person's neuromotor activity is to make the muscles on the right side of his body contract, taking his weight off of the left leg and onto the right. And we must remind ourselves that we are not looking at a static structure that, like a building, has sagged over onto its right side; on the contrary, we are looking at a living, moving human being, whose neural system is actively and at all times pulling his body over to the right. This neural one-sidedness is a condition that I have come to describe as somatic lateralization.

People who have shifted their weight over to their dominant side have a skeletomuscular system that is under considerable strain. If they are right-handed, the right side of their bodies is tightly compressed, and eventually this compression takes its toll. With many persons it is a pain in the right shoulder; in others the pain occurs in the neck on the right side. Sometimes the right ankle or knee will become weak and painful; for others there will be a soreness in the right side of the lumbar region. Often people will have a persistent headache in the right side of the head.

Charlie H. had an intense pain in his right hip joint. It had started some five years earlier, forcing him—an enthusiastic athlete—to give up all sports. Swimming was the only athletic activity he could do comfortably. He said that the medical diagnosis was that he had severely damaged the cartilage in his right hip joint. His orthopedic surgeon had suggested a surgical replacement of the hip joint. Instead, Charlie decided to have silicon injections in the joint, a procedure that relieved the pain for a while and then, when the pain began to return, he would have another injection. But after a certain number of these treatments, the silicon injections failed to work. When he first came to see me, he was in constant pain and walked with a heavy, rolling limp.

As Charlie stood facing me, he looked like a man who was being bent by a strong wind blowing from his left. His head was tilted far down on the right, the right shoulder was dropped a full two inches, and even the right side of his face was compressed. Also he had chronic headaches. He said that he was right-handed. I made some tests to see which leg he was standing on; it was the right. While he was still standing, I palpated the left and right sides of his spinal column. The muscles on the right side were like cable; those on the left side were soft. The right paravertebral muscles were contracted, curling the spine over to the right. Charlie was a perfect example of somatic lateralization.

To help him, I would have to find a way of changing his one-sidedness to two-sidedness—namely, to change his habit of standing on his right side and teach his muscular system to shift the body's weight over to the left leg. What Charlie was doing was wearing the hip joint down by making it support all of the weight of his upper body. Despite the fact that he was now crippled by his one-sided posture, it had never occurred to him to attempt to shift his weight over to the other foot. The invisible wind that ceaselessly bent him to one side was a wind that could not be felt: Charlie was unaware of his laterally bent posture.

Changing the way in which a person stands is not a simple matter, inasmuch as it involves the modification of hundreds of involuntary patterns of muscular contraction. One might think that it would be enough to look Charlie in the eye and say, "Charlie, stop leaning over on your right foot and stand straight!" I could have done this, but it would have been futile. Voluntarily and deliberately, Charlie could have leaned back onto his left side, but at the instant that he ceased to think about it, the involuntary contractions would immediately take charge again, pulling him firmly back to the right—and he would not even notice it. What needed to be done was to change these involuntary contractions so that, even when he was not thinking about it, he would automatically stand in vertical balance. This involved changing neither Charlie's volition nor even his muscles per se, but changing the neural impulses that innervated these muscles. When I looked at Charlie, what I saw was a distorted central nervous system.

Because Functional Integration is a complex art, it would be useless to attempt a description of the specific efforts that were made to change the patterns of his muscular contraction. For the moment, it is enough to say that my aim was to decrease the tonus of the muscles on the right side of his body and increase the tonus of those on the left. As soon as the muscle tension on the right side was decreased, ceasing to pull Charlie's trunk over to the right, his body would be free to return to a vertical stance. The hidden, autonomic operations of the sensorimotor system and the semicircular canals are such that if the body ceases to be pulled over to one side by involuntary contraction, it will once again reposition itself over the vertical line of gravity, very much in the way that a floating cork with a weighted bottom will pop back up to vertical if one ceases to push it over to the side.

Charlie began to pop back up, but not as quickly as a cork. It was careful and slow work, but after two sessions his headaches were gone and he was beginning to walk greater distances. He still limped, however, and the right-leaning posture and persistent pain continued, even though diminished. After the fourth session Charlie began to have days when he was completely pain-free. His face was now softer and longer on the right side, and the right eye was wider. Rather than being held high, the right side of the pelvis was down a bit, but he still tilted his head to the right and held his shoulder down.

It was time for some fine tuning, namely, a deliberate education of his faculties of self-sensing. I had Charlie stand with his eyes closed and begin rocking to the left and right from one foot to the other. I told him to rock to the right, then tilt back toward center until he felt that his head was vertical, and then continue past that point, rocking over to the left side. I watched him as he did this, and what happened was fascinating. I asked him, "Charlie, tell me each time you come past the vertical point. When you feel that your body is exactly straight up and down, let me know." Charlie did this, telling me each time when he felt that he was vertical. What was fascinating was that Charlie never once came up to a full vertical stance. He rocked back and forth purely on the right side, going from slightly right to far right.

A somatic distortion is not simply a distortion of the body's structure; it is a distortion of our awareness of ourselves in the physical world. In a certain sense, it is a distortion of our body image. Charlie's body image was so one-sided that he could no longer experience either bodily straightness or the relation of his body to gravity. A somatic distortion is a distortion of one's being—not of something called the mind nor of something called the body but of one's entire living being.

As one comes to observe the relationship between human function and human structure, knowing that the person before you has a conscious experience that, at the nonverbal level of sensorimotor functions, is constantly colored by these functional patterns, one comes to appreciate that the living reality experienced by human individuals is not in the least standardized. What is normal and usual in the experience of one individual may be radically different from what is normal to another individual. But neither of these two individuals will know just how different their "realities" are, because they have no basis of comparison. They always know only their own personal reality and no other. During the years of my work with others I have been repeatedly struck by the unavoidable evidence that a large number of people live a life of hell but do not realize that this is the case; instead, they consider their everyday pain, distortion, imbalance, and confusion as being the norm. Many times a client has suddenly looked at me and said, "Do you mean that I am *supposed* to feel comfortable?" This is always a person who has lived with distress and unhappiness for so long that he has no other expectation. After all, how could he know that any other experience is possible? We pass hundreds of our fellow men and women every day, all of them looking somewhat alike, and we assume that the experience of all these persons is the same. It is not. The conscious experience of different individuals is vastly and sometimes grotesquely different, but they will never know this, nor will anyone else.

Charlie had become a thoroughly one-sided human being. He was out of kilter with the world, because he had given up the use of one side of his life—his left side—and had invested everything in the more "intelligent" right side. If he were a boxer, he would have been a failure, because he would always have "led with his right," always going for the quick knockout punch. This was a simpleminded, one-sided approach to life, which belied the fact that Charlie was quite well educated. As the owner of an automotive dealership, he was successful with this simpleminded, one-punch tactic. But both in his personal life and in his physiological life, he was a cripple, incompetent to handle his family life, which was now in the shambles of divorce, and incompetent to handle his body, which had been moving toward a full breakdown.

All somatic distortions reflect problems that are simultaneously problems of the person's body and problems of the person's life-style. Within the context of the living functions of a human being, these two areas are inseparable. Viewed somatically, a human individual is neither a body nor a mind but, rather, a living, self-aware person with a single functional identity that shows itself in his awareness just as it shows itself in the functions of his body. This somatic vision, by focusing on the functional identity of a human being, reveals the integral and systemic nature of human individuality in a way that goes beneath the professional viewpoints of physiology and psychology. In learning to see people in this integral manner, one is at first startled by the transparent way in which "mental" ailments and "physical" ailments line up—as in binocular vision—to merge into a single, full-dimensional image.

Somatic distortions are functional distortions, and once we come to understand their serious significance, we realize that we have discovered the "no-man's land" of contemporary medicine and psychotherapy, namely, the realm of diseases that have no known cause and no known cure. Because the physician and psychotherapist tend to focus on the presumed "bodily" or "mental" components of the human being, respectively, they may fail to see the living, integral human individual who stands before them. Thus, they can see neither the "cause" of what is wrong nor the "cure."

The human soma is a functional system that will rebalance and reharmonize itself if given the chance. In functional disorders, what is required is not the exchange of words with the "mind," nor is it the exchange of chemicals and substances with the "body." The requirement is a change in the living human system's awareness of its own functioning. The somatic system needs more information of itself and more efficient control. In sum, the distorted human soma needs new sensory information and new motor control. As we go more deeply into this, I hope it will become transparently clear that our anciently evolved bodies would not have survived so long and so successfully without these internal abilities of self-balancing and self-correction. All somas have these abilities; it is only the human soma that represses these abilities through the process of acculturation and the attainment of "adulthood."

As Charlie became more aware of how he was actually functioning, he began to function better. As he began to sense when his body was distorted over to the right and when it was straight and in line with gravity, he began to stand straight, ceasing to limp and to be in pain. But this was not all. A somatic understanding tells us that such a sensorimotor change involves a change in consciousness—what psychologists might describe as a change in personality.

Charlie's "personality" did change. As he came upright, he also became aware of new things about himself. During one session he said, "You know, my wife is probably right.

I *am* insensitive." Charlie began reading books by Carl Jung. "You know," he said, "it makes sense that a man could spend the early part of his life developing only one aspect of his personality and not discover until middle age that there are other aspects that are equally part of him but that are totally undeveloped. That's the way I'm beginning to think about myself."

Beatrice S. had somewhat this same insight as she began to rediscover her balance. She was a first-rate journalist in her late twenties, who came to me because of severe pain in the right side of her neck. The neck pain had been chronic during the past four years and had become unbearable during the past few months. As can be expected with persons who have distortions of their somatic functions, she had initially been treated by various medical procedures, including neck braces, nerve block injections, and physical therapy, but this had no significant effect. Following that, she had tried chiropractic, then acupressure treatments, then relaxation training, then acupuncture—the gamut. Now she stood before me with her shoulders tensed upward in protection against the neck pain, her head pulled to the right, the left shoulder up and the right shoulder down, her torso bent, and her weight firmly planted on the right foot—and she was right-handed.

After two sessions, Beatrice reported that 50 percent of the pain had disappeared. When she came for the third session, she was standing almost vertical and she said that her left side felt stronger and more awake. After the fourth session, she told me that she was beginning to feel lighter on the right side and heavier on the left. This meant that she was becoming aware of the relaxation of muscles on the right side of her body and the gain in tonus of the muscles on the left.

During the sixth session she was feeling happy and comfortable, and it was at this time that she asked me a curious question. She said, "Does what you are doing have some kind of effect on my head? I mean, I've started to have all sorts of feelings and fantasies that are very literary and poetic. It's as if the artistic side of me is waking up."

I was delighted with this. I told her that her heavy right-sided dominance was not simply a physical event; rather it meant that she was using the left hemisphere of her brain almost to the exclusion of the right hemisphere. She was well read enough to know that recent brain research had uncovered the significant fact that the left hemisphere of the brain (which controls the right side of the sensorimotor functions of the body) is functionally different from the right. The left brain operates in logical, mathematical, verbal sequences, whereas the right side of the brain functions quite differently. It is best at grasping images, shapes, and whole units. The right hemisphere of the brain is, in many respects, the "artistic" side.

Modification of one's somatic functions is, simultaneously, modification of the entire living system. It is for this reason that the changes in Beatrice's body involved a change in Beatrice's life. Hers were not bodily improvements but somatic improvements. The unused portion of herself had become "awake" and "stronger," and she began to entertain different ideas about her future and what she wanted to do with her life. She was marvelously competent in her newspaper work, but she realized that, rewarding as it was, the kind of work she was doing was drudgery.

Beatrice had, like Charlie and many other persons I have worked with, discovered that she was not using all of herself. She had scaled down her way of living to a fine edge of competence, achieving a one-sided specialization. She had committed all of herself to the right side, abandoning the left as if it were useless—which is to say that she had been drawn into allowing the left hemisphere of her brain to tyrannize, as it were, the right-brain functions, firmly repressing them. This was a distortion of her body and of her life that she had been able to sustain for only a certain length of time before the entire system had begun to break down, sending her neck into painful spasm.

One thing can be said for those who develop a one-sided way of living: They are determined. Indeed, they are too determined; they are trying too hard. This is one of the most persistent personality traits of persons who are somatically lateralized. They are tenacious and willing to ignore and sacrifice much in order to achieve excellence. What they sacrifice is one half of their organic being. They have sacrificed their wholeness. Certainly there is a kind of desperation and "driven" quality to this way of being, an overevaluation of the recognition, the money, or the power that they seek to achieve. Somatically, one-sided human beings are, I find, "good people" with a ferocious commitment to achievement. With their "one-punch" approach to their task, they can be pointedly effective, but little do they realize how weak is their overall ability to live successfully.

As they come toward balance and lose their one-sidedness, these people become far more powerful and far more competent as human beings. They become more confident and clear-headed about who they are and where they are in relation to the rest of the world, so that, balanced and fully functioning, when they take aim at something, they do not miss the mark.

Somatic retraction, somatic fixation, and somatic lateralization—all of these are distortions of the spatiality of the human soma. All three are distortions of something so ancient and so obvious that it is astonishing to realize that what we have been speaking of all along are the three dimensions of space: length, depth, and width.

Commentary: The Function of Handling

Some features of life are so elemental that they seem mysterious. For example, take something as simple and commonplace as the way a mirror reflects the image of our bodies. As we stand before the glass, there before us is the mirror image of ourselves, perfect in every respect except that the right side is on the left and the left side is on the right. The reversal of the two sides is so familiar to us that it might never occur to us to ask a curious question: Why doesn't the image reverse top to bottom and bottom to top, just as it does the two sides?

Is it the mirror that creates this oddity? Is it, perhaps, some peculiarity in the angles of light reflection? Is it something about our visual perception? Or is it something else?

The truth is that we know the answer to this puzzle, but it is so much below the threshold of our consciousness that we may never have articulated it. The reason that the mirror reverses our two sides but not our top and bottom has to do neither with the mirror nor with the light nor with our visual perception. It has to do with the nature of our bodily structure: We are bilaterally symmetrical.

Our mirror image has an invisible vertical line that comes straight down through the middle of our body, revealing two identical sides. Our bodies are designed with a vertical line of symmetry, creating two halves that look interchangeably the same. But between the top and bottom of our bodies there is no horizontal line of symmetry, nor is there any identity between the upper and lower halves. Bilateral symmetry is not simply a human fact, it is a somatic fact: All living things tend to have two identical vertical sides.

Or roughly identical. Looked at closely, the two sides of the human body are not exactly the same. The heart is not in the middle; it is on the left side, which means that the left lung is smaller than the right. The stomach and pancreas are also on the left side, whereas the liver and appendix are on the right. It appears that life strives to be almost perfectly symmetrical but not quite. This, in itself, is significant, as we shall soon discover.

We do not need a mirror to discover that one side of our body is the mirror image of the other; we need only look. But in looking, we should keep in mind that a mirror image is a *reversed* image, like turning a sheet of carbon paper backward when drawing a picture. The carbon copy is, in every detail, exactly like the original, except that it is in reverse. If you have written *mud* on the original, the reversed carbon will say *bum.* If the hair is parted on the left, the carbon will show it parted on the right. The rings on the left hand appear on the right hand in the mirror image. So it takes a moment's reflection to realize that mirror-image identity is not, after all, identical. As full proof of this, we can take a frontal picture of a human body, cut with scissors right down the middle line of symmetry, then throw away the left side, keeping the right side only. We can then make a photostatic copy of the right side, so that we have two sides—two absolutely identical right sides. When we take the two sides and put them together to make a whole human being, they won't match. With two absolutely identical sides we cannot make a whole human being for the same reason that with two identical letter *c*'s we cannot make an *o* unless we turn one *c* around to form a *ɔ*. What is lacking is mirror-image identity, with one side coming to the center line from the right and another side coming to the center line from the left.

It looks as if life makes its bodies out of two mirror-image halves that are put together along the vertical line of symmetry. Since that seems to be the case, we know automatically that bilateral symmetry is built into the genetic information by which bodies are constructed. Curious evidence of this is found in twins, who sometimes each have asymmetric features that go one way in one twin and the other way in the other twin. In Siamese twins this mirror imaging is dramatic: One is right-handed while the other is left-handed; if the cowlick of one twin's hair spins clockwise, the other's spins counterclockwise; the fingerprints of one twin's right hand will be nearest to matching not his own left hand but the left hand of the other. But we don't see the full extent of this mirror imaging until we notice that one Siamese twin always has "transposed viscera." The internal organs are reversed: The heart is on the right, the liver is on the left, and so on.

Therefore, all somas have two more or less identical sides, just as all somas stand upright and all somas face into the world. *More or less* does not imply exact identity. As biological inquirers, as soon as we know that the two sides are not structurally identical, we are awake to the probability that neither are they functionally identical. As we know, this is the case. The two sides do not operate in the same way—particularly in human beings.

In animals other than human beings, there is no functional preference of one side over the other. A bird may perch on a favored leg, even as a dog may point with a particular leg, but there is no general right-handedness or left-handedness in nonhuman animals. Even in our nearest evolutionary ancestors, there is no species preference; monkeys and apes do not have a specific dominance of one hand over the other.

It is only in ourselves that lateral dominance is a genetic fact, and this should alert us to the possibility that dominant-handedness is a significant trait of the human species. Not all humans are right-handed, but the overwhelming majority are. Studies have been made of pictorial and other signs of hand dominance cross-culturally, covering a period of five thousand years. The results are that, at least since 3,000 B.C., roughly 92.6 percent of humans have had right-hand dominance.

Left-handers have always been a small minority, living in a world where everything from doorknobs to handshakes is right-handed. If the left-hander is Chinese or Japanese or Israeli, he will luckily be able to read books in the way he finds easiest, from right to left. Otherwise, he must put up with wristwatches, telephone booths, pencil sharpeners, and egg beaters that are not designed with him in mind. And he must put up with ancient linguistic traditions that imply—not so subtly—that *right* and *droit* and *recht* mean "correct," "lawful," and "just" to English, French, and Germans, respectively. And that left-handers are linguistically accused of being "sinister," "awkward," "crooked," and, perhaps, "evil."

In earlier decades the sinistral minority was believed to be defective in serious ways. Stammering, it was once theorized, is caused by forcing a left-handed child to become right-handed. This was also presumed to bring on emotional difficulties. A century ago a psychiatrist named Cesare Lombroso added righteous insult to injury by suggesting that left-handedness was a sign of criminal degeneracy. All of these theories are nonsense, but they illustrate how a predominantly right-handed world has skeptically viewed the beleaguered clan of lefties.

For their part, left-handers frequently suspect that the dextrous majority is secretly envious of the superiority of the sinistral minority. After all, one need only look at the number of left-handed athletes celebrated in the sports world. This theory is, however, as baseless as the heavy-handed theories of the righties. There is no question that the lefty can perform as well as his lateral counterpart, but it is not the case that he is superior. What advantage he may have in the sports world is completely tied up with the fact that right-handers do not know how to handle him. When a star left-handed hitter comes to bat in a clutch inning, the manager makes a most practical move: He sends in a left-handed pitcher. Being more concerned with success than with theory, managers and coaches know very well that handedness gives no superiority unless the opposing athlete has the opposite handedness.

So, athletes and all other somas have bilateral symmetry

(more or less), and depending on dominance, one side can function just as well as the other. If we wish to go more deeply into this rather mysterious subject of bilaterality, we need to look more deeply into living bodies, especially at the brain.

In all vertebrate creatures (i.e., fish, amphibians, reptiles, birds, and mammals) there is bilateral symmetry in the brain: One side is identical with the other. At first this doesn't seem surprising, until we look more closely at the structure of the vertebrate brain and see that it is not simply one brain but, rather, is comprised of two identical hemispheres that are joined together. We vertebrates do not have one brain but two brains in tandem, joined at the vertical line of symmetry.

The fact of two hemispheres of the cerebral cortex has always fascinated brain researchers. Those two halves of gray matter are joined together at one point by millions of tough white fibers that relay information from one hemisphere to the other, so that the hemispheres can coordinate with each other. These fibers are called the corpus callosum.

Thus there arose the question, What would happen if the corpus callosum was surgically cut, thus splitting the two identical brain hemispheres? Would all coordination disappear? Would the animal be totally disoriented or, possibly, destroyed? Therefore, an experiment was performed back in the 1950s upon a cat, whose corpus callosum was neatly severed. Following the operation the cat seemed normal, so the researchers devised a way of seeing just how normal a cat it was. They put a patch over one of the cat's eyes, which meant that what the cat saw would go to only one hemisphere; the other hemisphere, because of the surgery, would not pick up the information.

Looking like a feline pirate, the cat with its eye patch was put into a laboratory box where there were two little swinging doors. Behind one door was food; behind the other was a nozzle that would immediately blow out an irritating puff of air if its door was pushed. It did not take the cat long to learn which door to push and which door to avoid: It always went to the door with food.

Then the cat was removed from the box, and its patch was switched to the other eye. Nothing else was done to the cat. The cat, now looking through its opposite eye for the first time, was put back into the box. Since the cat had already learned which door held the food, it could be expected to head straight for the food door, but it did not. It acted as if it had never before been in the box, nor did it know which door was which. It blundered into the door with the puff of air, just as if it had never learned anything.

This strange event led the experimenters to try something else. They switched the doors, putting the food behind the puff-of-air door and moving the nozzle over to where the food had been. The cat, still wearing its opposite patch, quickly learned to deal with this situation. Now it went to the other door for its food, avoiding the puff of air.

Then, leaving the box in this same state, they simply took the cat out and switched the patch back to the original eye. It was as if it were another cat. It kept going to the wrong door. But whenever they switched the eye patch back, it suddenly knew very well which door to go to. They discovered that with the patch on one eye, the cat could learn one door system, and then with the patch on the opposite eye, it could learn the reversed door system; but the two learnings never connected. There were, effectively, two cats: the right-eyed cat, who knew one thing,

and the left-eyed cat, who knew the opposite thing. But the right-eyed cat had no knowledge of the left-eyed cat. This was an unsettling result. It appeared that there were two cats occupying the same body, each one able to take total control in its own way and with its own personality.

Then the scary question presented itself, If the corpus callosum was severed in a human being, would this mean that there would be two separate personalities, one not knowing what the other was doing? Does bilateral symmetry of the brain mean that we are two separate beings somehow joined together? An unsettling question, indeed, which, one would think, had little possibility of being answered. But it soon was.

In 1960 Dr. Joseph Bogen, of Los Angeles, suggested a way in which severe epilepsy could be controlled. A thorough review of the research literature indicated that the out-of-phase left-right hemispheric disturbance typical of epileptics could, in many instances, be controlled by severing the corpus callosum. The first person to be so helped by this surgical procedure was studied by Bogen, Michael Gazzaniga, and Roger W. Sperry during the early 1960s, Sperry being one of the persons who had done the earlier experiments with cats. The first publication of their observations alerted the scientific community that a new chapter had begun in brain research.

Their initial observations confirmed what the cat experiments had found in the 1950s: Information coming into one hemisphere—visual, tactile, proprioceptive, auditory, and olfactory—was responded to by that hemisphere without the other hemisphere having any awareness of it. The information did not transfer.

Further studies of this patient revealed that despite

his apparent composure and normal behavior, there were some amazing differences between the way the two hemispheres functioned. Given their neat separation, one could observe the functions of each brain hemisphere in its purity, so to speak. So observed, it suddenly became apparent that the two hemispheres were not symmetrically the same in their functions but were radically different.

As you may remember, sense data coming into the right eye or right hand is generally routed to the opposite side of the brain, the left hemisphere. The same criss-cross pattern occurs in the case of information coming into the left visual field and the left hand. In one test, the patient was shown a word, such as *spoon,* in his left visual field (right hemisphere) and was then asked what he saw. He replied that he had not seen anything. But then, when his left hand was given a number of objects to examine, among them a spoon, he immediately recognized it. He neither knew the word nor could he verbally recognize it in print, but his right hemisphere knew the shape and texture of *spoon.* Of course, if they flashed the word *spoon* in his right visual field, he immediately knew and recognized the word.

Long before these experiments, it was known that the left brain hemisphere is centrally involved in language, but it was not known to what extent. Bogen and his fellow researchers discovered that language, counting, and analytical thinking are specialties of the left hemisphere almost exclusively. The right hemisphere, in contrast, is nearly totally lacking in linguistic abilities.

Because the abilities of the right side of the brain are nonverbal, special experiments had to be devised to tease out the nature of these abilities. Here are some of the right-hemispheric talents that have been catalogued: The right hemisphere is crucial for spatial orientation. If the right side of the brain is damaged, a person will easily become lost; he can neither use nor draw maps; he misjudges the size, distance, and direction of objects; he cannot copy simple shapes accurately or draw slanted lines properly; he will not recognize faces, nor can he remember unfamiliar or unusual shapes. This peculiarity is not confined to vision but is the same for the sense of touch and the sense of hearing. Right-brain damage diminishes a human being's ability to recognize melodies and chords.

An important finding in hemispheric brain research is that one side of the brain is not simply "dominant" over the other; rather, each side has a specialization. If a split-brain patient is asked to describe something verbally, his left hemisphere does the job automatically; if he is asked to locate something, his right hemisphere springs into operation, and the patient points with his finger.

The human brain appears to be structurally symmetrical, but it is radically asymmetrical in its functions. We have two ways of knowing things, two different kinds of intelligence. In some instances one kind is more useful; at other times the other is more useful. These contrasting left-brain/right-brain ways of processing information have been expressed by means of the following generalities:

symbolic/spatial
analytic/synthetic
rational/metaphoric
active/receptive
abstract/concrete

linear / nonlinear
sequential / multiple

After fifteen years of sifting through these contrasts, Joseph Bogen believes that the most accurate way of contrasting left- and right-hemisphere functions is "propositional" versus "appositional." To "propose" is to put forward assertively; to "appose" is to fit with and adapt to. Together they constitute the warp and woof of cognition and thinking.

More specifically, Bogen's mature understanding of these differences involves a distinction in terms of *time:* The left hemisphere organizes things temporally. Years of experimentation support this view that the left side processes things one-by-one in sequence, whereas the right side can process complex information all at once at the same instant. The left brain's secret is a linear temporal sequence. The right brain's secret is a nonlinear, nontemporal, simultaneous grasping of a total configuration.

Research in hemispheric differences continues at a fascinating pace, but enough has been confirmed to teach us that symmetry of the two sides has, in the human species, been both violated and transcended. There is no doubt that asymmetry is biologically advantageous and that the human being has evolved to use this advantage. Whereas the apes are ambidextrous, the vast majority of humans are, and apparently always have been, predominantly right-handed—and also right-eyed, right-footed, and even right-jawed in chewing.

Human beings do not deal with problems using both hands. They are more selective. They use one hand and one side in order to perform in a more specialized way.

Human beings, like all somas, have advanced in efficiency and complexity through a basic biological device: differentiation. That is what human laterality is, *a differentiation of function that automatically creates two discrete functions.*

Because there is an ancient, invisible line of vertical symmetry dividing the structure of all somas, somas have an option in the way they can manage things from one side or the other. That is a convenience, because it gives the soma double the options in its maneuvering. *Manage* and *maneuver* both stem from the same Latin word: *manus,* meaning "hand." We have seen that the first function of somas is *to stand upright;* the second is *to face;* and the third primordial function is *to handle.*

All somas have ways of handling the world. Usually, these ways are random and not species-specific, but in the human soma, the two sides of the body and the two sides of the brain are bilaterally specialized. (And in most instances, there are minor structural differences in the left hemisphere's "speech area.") Here we have touched upon something of, possibly, enormous consequence. Consider the facts: (1) human beings are the only creatures to have evolved into lateral specialization; (2) human beings are the only creatures who use language, which nearly always operates through the left hemisphere. These are not simple coincidences: *Language is a specialized way in which the human species handles the world.*

One of the most helpful ways of visualizing the peculiar fact of human asymmetry and lateral specialization is the image of an archer. The archer uses both hands. The left holds the wood of the bow and the arrow tip; the right holds the string and the arrow's base. Both sides and both hands function together, each performing its special task. The right foot and side are planted; they are the stable center of action. The left foot and hand are extended outward from this center, rotating and adjusting the aim so that the arrow can line up between the eye and its intended target. The archer's left side (right hemisphere) adjusts the body internally until the aim is true. Holding the string is the right hand, positioned just under the right eye, and almost touching the mouth and cheek. The aiming and firing of the arrow is a bilateral action: The left side adjusts internally to line up eye-arrow-target; the right eye and hand remain fixed and centered, judging the exact instant when the left side has been lined up with eye and target.

Then the arrow is released. Just like a soma moving headlong into the world, its trajectory is corrected and aimed by the efficient coordination of two very different hands.

This coordination of two different sides and two specialized functions is a more efficient way for the human being to operate. Two specialized functions integrated into a single coordinated process is what the timing function is made to accomplish. If it lost one of those specialized functions, the soma would diminish in efficiency and become lateralized. The chapter on somatic lateralization showed the consequences of investing all of one's effort into a one-sided stance. Eventually the body breaks down, and one's self-image is severely imbalanced, so much so that one can no longer live effectively and comfortably.

The two sides of the human soma are different, and we are fortunate to have this difference. It adds richness to our experience and our actions. We may encourage the further development of this difference between our two sides, knowing that a superior neural function guarantees their integration. The timing function synthesizes these differences, blending them into the regular repertoire of our larger system of moving and sensing.

The two sides of life are separate but equal; together, they allow us to handle the world in ways that are easy and effective. If we stand before our mirror, looking at these two sides for long enough, we may discover a secret. When we wondered why the mirror reversed the image of our two sides but not our top and bottom, we were not quite accurate. The mirror does *not* reverse the two sides. Our left side still remains on the left side of the mirror, and our right side remains on the right. Nothing has changed or switched. What we see is a perfect reflection of ourselves, with each of our sides retaining its same position.

But, then, why is it that almost all of us look at ourselves in the mirror and see our two sides reversed? The answer has to do with our culture and the way in which it makes us focus outward upon the bodily structure of other individuals. We think that the image in the mirror has reversed its sides because, without realizing it, we assume that we are looking at someone else, at another person standing in front of us. Our culture so externalizes our perception that, even when looking at ourselves, we absentmindedly assume that what we see is a body other than our own. It is not. What we see is ourself, our own body, whose left side is supposed to be on the left and whose right side is supposed to be on the right. There never was a reversal; we merely had the illusion that there was a reversal.

This is how our culture distorts our perception. We cannot see ourselves for what we are. To assume that our mirror image is someone else is a sign that our sense of personal identity is externalized and that our internal sense of identity is atrophied. It all depends on how we look at ourselves. Try it yourself. Look in a mirror. Are your sides reversed, or do they remain on the same side? The answer will tell you how well you know yourself.

2 / temporal distortion of the living body

SOMATIC INEFFICIENCY

For a karate expert to break a two-inch board with the side of his hand, it requires timing. A complex sequence of muscular contractions takes place: The diaphragm contracts violently, expelling air; all of the flexor muscles in the front of the body contract, forcing the legs heavily downward and bringing the torso forward and downward; this forward curling of the trunk does not happen all at once but in successive contractions of powerful muscles around the spine, triggering the contraction of one vertebra after the other in a rising chain of innervations, climaxed by the sequential dropping of the shoulder blade, then the forearm, then the wrist. This movement, beginning with the heavy, powerful muscles in the pelvis, radiates upward in ever-increasing speed and rising force until the final velocity and power of the culminating blow become devastating.

When a man takes a rock or a baseball, lifts one leg, arches his back, whips his spine forward, and releases the object—which has suddenly accelerated from a speed of zero to a speed of nearly one hundred miles per hour—this, too, is a matter of timing. When a tennis player brings his racket forward, turning waist, shoulder, elbow, and wrist to strike the oncoming ball with a smooth, almost effortless *thong,* it is a matter of timing. When Horowitz or Menuhin put their hands to their instruments before a thousand eager listeners, it is their sense of timing that brings forth the audience's enraptured applause.

There is something quite magical about timing; when we see human timing at its peak of efficiency, we are awed and uplifted. It reminds us of the extraordinary possibilities of ourselves as human beings. It also reminds us that without efficient timing of our actions, our lives are clumsy and ineffectual. But the martial arts, the athletic arts, and the performing arts are merely special instances of timing. Timing itself is not special. It is a defining characteristic of every action of every living creature from its inception to its death. Specifically, timing is the function of integrating all three spatial dimensions of the body in simultaneous movement.

The three types of somatic distortion we have mentioned all involve deformations of the longitudinal, profunditudinal, and latitudinal directions of somatic movement. All living beings have six bodily segments that we recognize as distinctive and characteristic features of living, moving bodies. The two ends of the length of a soma are not the same; rather, they are distinguished as head and tail, as the superior-rostral end and the inferior-caudal end. Likewise, in their depth somas have a face and a back, otherwise referred to as the anterior-ventral portion and the posterior-dorsal portion. And in their width, all somas have two distinctive sides, one that is to the left of the middle line and one that is to the right.

Considered as segments of a dead, unmoving body, the dimensions of length, depth, and width are static, geometrical positions. But somas are not dead; they are moving, and because of this constant movement, these three dimensions are not simply spatial coordinates, they are three distinct spatial functions. All living beings, even amoebas, tend to lengthen in forward motion, the head end is the end that "heads into" the environing world. Thus, one of the soma's functions is to lengthen. Inversely, one of its malfunctions would be a chronic shortening of this length, and this is what I have called somatic retraction. All somas have a face, which is not merely a static coordinate but, in life, involves a constantly changing position. To live, move, and survive, a soma must be able to face in any direction it needs, and a malfunction of facing is what I have called somatic fixation, that is, the chronic inability to face in all directions. All somas have two sides, and from their outer body inward to their neural centrum they have the functional ability to move both toward the left side and toward the right side. Inability to perform both of these lateral functions is what I have termed somatic lateralization. Although we have illustrated these three functional dimensions in reference to ourselves, the human species, all three are characteristic of the bodily functions of all living creatures. By the same token, all other creatures can suffer these same malfunctions.

All too frequently the most difficult thing to see and understand is the obvious. This is, and always has been, the challenge of authentic philosophizing: seeing and understanding that which is elemental and fundamental. In introducing this book, I remarked that the question What is life? is, taken abstractly, unanswerable, but if this question is posed in concrete terms—by looking at living bodies, the sole bearers of life—then the question can be answered. What I have done is to develop this answer in very concrete terms, by pointing out those specific malfunctions in human beings that have the dual quality of being quite common and yet quite mysterious. Anytime we encounter something with the dual quality of being both commonplace and yet inscrutable, we know that we have come face to face with a matter that, most likely, is elemental and fundamental. In the last chapter I sought to bring these elemental features to light, and what seems to have been revealed is something so obvious that one wonders how anyone could have been so inattentive as not to notice it. This is the discovery that at the core of all living beings—including ourselves—are the three dimensions of space. In order for life to exist at all in this universe, the body of life had—in its very constitution—to incorporate the three dimensions of physical space into its functions as well as its structure.

All living creatures are three-dimensional in both structure and function, and when we contemplate the complexity of inwardly controlling and mobilizing all three dimensions, we should be surprised that it is even possible. Mobilizing a body for movement involves ordering the whole body into a coordinated, fluidly adjusting trajectory. This is possible only by means of a single agency of control that is capable of mobilizing all portions of the soma to a single task. This controlling agency is supplied by the cen-

tral nervous system. It is the function of timing, sequential coordination of the whole organism in a u action. The timing function guarantees the interna ciency of the living body. It can do this because it i function of the central nervous system that integrate of our muscular movements and sensory awareness simultaneous action.

We are seldom aware of the extraordinarily watchfu and efficient operations of the timing function. When we perform any voluntary action, such as lifting one foot, we usually fail to notice the unified, mobilizing action of the entire body. At this moment, if you are sitting, you can demonstrate this for yourself by lifting the right foot off the floor for a few seconds and then putting it down again. Normally, when we perform a deliberate action such as this, our awareness is focused on the foot as it leaves the floor and then returns to it. But if one continues this simple movement and focuses one's attention on other parts of one's body, some remarkable things will be noticed. For example, when the right foot lifts, what is happening under the left side of the pelvis and under the left thigh? For that matter, what is the left foot doing when the right foot is lifting? Is it, too, rising, or is it, instead, pressing down? You may notice that, quite apart from your conscious intention to lift the right foot, there is an automatic and unconscious mobilization of the left leg to press downward. It is not you who are deliberately pressing down the left leg; it is your timing function, which mobilizes the whole of your body in coordination with your intended movement. As you continue lifting the right foot and setting it down, let your awareness come upward to your right shoulder. Is it slightly moving? If so, in which direc-

tion is it moving when you lift the right foot? Once you've determined this, bring your internal awareness over to the left shoulder. Can you detect any movement there? In which direction? If you are very attentive, you may notice that when you lift the right foot, you are also slightly lifting the right shoulder and simultaneously dropping the left shoulder a bit. In fact, the deliberate lifting of your right foot quietly causes the timing function to organize your whole body, so that the entire right side of the body lifts while the entire left side drops down and contracts. You may also notice that the muscles along the left side of the spine contract, bringing your weight over to the left, making a ballast on the left side to compensate for the extra weight of holding up the right foot.

This is what the timing function is doing all the time—in human bodies and in all living bodies. Consciously we may intend only a movement of one part of our bodies, but unconsciously the timing function coordinates the whole of the body, making that movement more efficient and thereby relieving the body of unneeded strain. It is all rather reassuring. Whether we even know it or not, our genes have given us a watchful, all-controlling function, whose purpose is to make our lives easier.

Looked at functionally, timing is a single, unified control that pervades the entire bodily system, integrating the three lower functions of standing, facing, and handling. Looked at anatomically, however, we see many different structures involved. For one thing, there is the vestibular system lodged in the mastoid bone just behind our ears, an organ whose three semicircular canals automatically control muscular contraction throughout the body. When someone suddenly slips on icy pavement, the vestibular

system reacts with lightninglike rapidity, bringing the body back into vertical balance long before our conscious attention has had any chance to respond. Another organ of the timing function is the cerebellum, a small, beautiful structure located just under the back of the brain and looking, for all the world, like a little replica of the brain. The cerebellum, with its left and right hemispheres, coordinates and balances the muscles of the whole body, making sure that when, for example, the right foot is lifted, the left foot presses down. This it does in cooperation with the vestibular system, which is concerned to keep the body in vertical alignment with the ever-present guideline of gravity. Other ingenious mechanisms in the spinal column make sure that when we contract a muscle, bringing a limb up in one direction, the antagonist muscle on the opposite side of the limb relaxes and extends. When we flex our biceps, showing how strong we are, we don't think to relax the triceps on the bottom of the upper arm; it happens automatically by reciprocal innervation, a special arrangement of circuitry between the spinal column and the muscles. There is much more of the central nervous system involved in the timing function, notably the cerebral cortex—that complex, neural super-computer that can program itself to learn the most complex things, such as breaking boards in two with a bare hand, throwing a ball ninety-five miles an hour, or playing a Chopin scherzo.

Considered structurally, then, the timing function is varied and complex, but considered in terms of its function, it is simple and unified, and it works to make all our movements efficiently coordinated, whether we are aware of it or not. However, we know already that this is not always the case. As these various case histories have indicated, it is common for people, especially those who are more highly civilized, to become painfully inefficient and clumsy in movement and in self-sensing. Despite its watchfulness and despite its pervasive control, the function of timing often fails in its task, not necessarily because of some fault in itself but because of some distortion, such as an habitual retraction of the body's length, a fixation of its ability to turn, or a one-sided lateralization away from the midline of the body. When any of these somatic distortions are present, the timing function is less efficient; its quiet, unconscious mobilizing power attempts to balance the body's movements but, given what it has to work with, it falls short of the mark. You will recall Charlie's attempt to lean to the left when his eyes were closed. He could not do so. Because he had been so long distorted over to the right side, the timing function was ludicrously ineffective in balancing his body. Also recall the banker whose spine was so fixated that when he thought he was rotating it, there was no visible movement whatsoever. The timing function cannot aid our intention to move in certain ways if one or more of the spatial dimensions of our bodies are distorted. Even though it is a higher, integrative function of the central nervous system, it can integrate only those sensorimotor patterns that it is given.

If we leave aside, for the moment, accidents of congenital deformity or physical injury, there are two basic factors that bring about somatic inefficiency: first, habitual somatic distortion; and, second, a deficiency in learning. It is encouraging to realize that both problems can be solved by the same general procedures, namely, becoming aware of oneself in the course of experiencing certain movements.

This procedure can be most appropriately illustrated by the cases of two professional musicians with whom I have worked: Pete R., a vibraphone player, and Martin J., who played the double bass.

For a year Pete had suffered chronic pain in his left wrist, with occasional and less intense pain in the right wrist. The vibraphone is a percussion instrument, somewhat like a marimba, that is played with either one or two mallets in each hand. Pete's left wrist was always painful; at the time we first met, he was unable to perform. During the year, he had received medical treatment for the wrist. Braces were helpful when he was not performing, but they interfered with his playing, so he would leave them off at those times. The day after a performance the wrist would be intensely sore again, brace or no brace. Then a physician recommended cortisone injections. Pete told me that the wrist responded to this by becoming more painful. Then an orthopedic specialist placed Pete's wrist in a brace, holding it immobile for two months in a backward, extended position. This made the wrist still more painful. X rays showed no structural damage in the wrist, and so it was a mystery why there should be so much pain.

When I examined Pete, exploring the way his body moved, I was struck by the immobility of his trunk. He was a small man, well-muscled and tightly erect: There was almost no rotation in the spine—it was fixated. The shoulder blades, as well, seemed cemented into the trunk, especially the left scapula, which allowed only the smallest movement. It took just a few minutes to see the functional problem: Pete swung his mallets purely with the motions of his wrist and elbow; there seemed to be no movement whatsoever of the shoulder blade and back. It was clear that the muscles of the wrist were painfully overworked after a standard performance of three hours' total playing time.

With Pete lying in various positions—on his stomach, back, and either side—I made small movements of his vertebrae, ribs, and shoulder blades, calling his attention to the sensations he felt as I did so. Bit by bit the movements of the torso began to be more differentiated; Pete could back up the movements of his forearm by adding to them the movements of his shoulder blades. Gradually, as I had him practice on an imaginary vibraphone, he began to turn his torso, rotating his spine sinuously all the way down to his hip joints and playing his imaginary instrument with his entire body. As the somatic fixation melted, there was more of Pete available to perform, and as this fuller movement developed, the expected result occurred: The pain in the wrist disappeared.

I should call attention to the fact that I did not do a medical feat of "curing" Pete by "removing the symptom" of pain in his wrist; on the contrary, I educated Pete by helping him to add more movement to his playing. If one considered Pete's problem from a structural viewpoint, then the focus would have been on his wrist. This was the nature of his earlier diagnosis and treatment. But if one considered Pete's problem from a somatic viewpoint, viewing his entire body in terms of its functions, then the focus was on everywhere *except* his wrist. As it was, I never touched his wrist, since that was not where the problem was; instead, I touched the rest of his body, reminding him of the parts he was not moving. Once they began moving, the timing function integrated these new movements—and new sensations—into the way in which he played the vibraphone.

When one deals with functionally caused problems in the proper manner—that is, functionally—there is no problem of getting rid of the pain; this is assumed as a matter of course. But my intention was far in advance of this. I wanted to help him become more aware and more in control of himself so that he could play the vibraphone better than he had before. And in this I succeeded—or rather we succeeded together.

My way of working with Martin J., the bass player, was much more obviously an educational procedure. Martin played the bass in a jazz band, using the index and middle fingers to pluck the strings. Each finger would, in quick succession, flex downward to pluck the string, then extend upward as the other finger flexed. It was a fast action, and during the past year Martin noticed that the entire length of a muscle in the back of his right forearm was becoming "weakened." Eventually each time he played, the muscle would become so painful that it would take a week of recovery before he could play again. That was when he came to see me.

He told me the situation, and I asked him to show me the muscle that was always so weak and painful. It was the *extensor communis digitorum,* which surprised me. I had thought that it would be the flexor movement of plucking the thick strings that caused the soreness; instead, it was the extensor movement of pulling the index and middle fingers away from the string with this extensor muscle.

I requested that Martin bring his bass with him for our second session so that I could see how he held the instrument and played it. He showed me. He would lean back on a high stool, sitting on the left side of his pelvis, his back rotated to the left as he hunched forward over the long arm of the bass. He played for me. Much like Pete, he played using only the two fingers, the wrist, and the elbow; the rest of his body was frozen in a curled position. But, unlike Pete, the rest of his body was not rigid or fixated; it was relatively supple. His was a different problem. Rather than a somatic distortion, Martin had a learning problem.

If Martin had been taught to play the bass in the traditional manner, I doubt that he would have run into any difficulty. When learning to play with a bow, the shoulder blade and spine are automatically called into a swaying, lateral movement by the bowing action. As it was, he was self-taught. He had borrowed a bass and learned to play it, fiercely focusing on his fingers and the strings, with the remainder of his body left out of the learning experience. Thus, when he became adept enough to become professional, the nightly performances taxed the use of his *extensor communis digitorum* beyond its capacity. My conclusion was that Martin had learned to play the bass in the wrong way. He had to be retaught.

I proposed an experiment to Martin. "Imagine," I said, "that your entire hand and elbow are paralyzed. Hold the two fingers out as if they are frozen and let the wrist and elbow be rigid." Martin did this. "Now I want you to play the bass by moving the arm with the shoulder blade."

Martin reflected on this a moment and then began to move the rigid arm. He brought the fingers down and laid the index finger beneath the string and plucked, then he dropped the shoulder blade, moved the arm forward again, and placed the middle finger beneath the string and plucked upward. He practiced this for a while, and soon he could manipulate the forearm and hand rather well. He was pleased; he had never thought of playing in this manner.

"You see," I commented, "if your forearm and hand actually *were* paralyzed, that still wouldn't prevent you from playing the bass. All a person needs to do is to bring another part of the body into action. There are people whose hands are paralyzed or deformed who learn to write and draw pictures with their feet. Compared with them, our feet seem paralyzed because they are so clumsy at doing carefully controlled movements. But if we had to, we could learn to write and draw with our feet; then they wouldn't seem so paralyzed. In a way, everyone's body has sections that are 'paralyzed,' simply because they have never learned to move those sections with any skill."

Once Martin could play with ease, using his shoulder blade for the movement, we went on to a second experiment. "Now, imagine that both your shoulder blade and your forearm-wrist are paralyzed. Play the bass using your spine and hip joints."

At first, of course, Martin's movements were clumsy; his overall coordination was inefficient. That only lasted a short while. Soon he was thumping the strings quite well, the strong muscles of the lower back and hips moving the "paralyzed" limbs adroitly.

Now we went to the next step. "Unfreeze the right shoulder blade and play, using the shoulder as well as the back and hip." As soon as he did this, he was playing easily and smoothly. Despite the "paralyzed" forearm-wrist, there was very little clumsiness in his movements.

The final step was for Martin to unfreeze the forearm

and begin using the elbow, wrist, and fingers once again, this time in coordination with the shoulders and lower back. Now with all of these parts moving together, Martin moved with grace and ease. From that moment onward, Martin ceased to have any pains in the back of the forearm. This was possible because he was now using all of himself to play. He had now learned something that had become a working part of his repertoire of movements. He would not forget how to do it.

One of the most frequent questions asked me by those whom I have helped to regain movement is, "But will it last? Won't the old condition come back again?" Martin asked me this. I said, "Well, the way you are playing now is something you learned, isn't it?" He admitted that this was the case. "Once you've learned a sequence of movements, you will find that you can't forget it. At this point, you can't help but play the bass with your whole body, because it's easier that way and because it sounds better. "Look," I asked, "how long ago did you learn to snap your fingers?" "Probably twenty years ago," he said. "And when," I asked, "was the last time you snapped your fingers?" He thought about it and realized that it had been a long time; in fact, he rarely, if ever, snapped his fingers anymore. "Then snap your fingers for me." He lifted his hand and snapped his fingers. "There's your answer," I said. "You can't forget how to snap your fingers, and you can't forget how to play the bass with your whole body. Once learned, it's too late to forget it; you are stuck with the skill you have learned, just as you were stuck with the inefficient way in which you first learned to play. If, for the rest of your life, you try to forget how to snap your fingers, you will never succeed. It is the same thing with the bass.

You may, for want of practice, play badly, but you won't ever be able to play without using the more efficient sequence of movements you have now learned."

I should add a third example, one not having to do with music but with athletics. In this case it was a counselor, who had suffered severe spasms in his lower back, so severe that he had fainted and was rushed off to a hospital. Counselors, psychotherapists, and psychiatrists are frequent visitors to my office, because of the sustained and heavy stress they must endure listening to the emotional problems of others. As illustrated in chapter 1, the typical muscular response to stress is somatic retraction, or, more specifically, a contraction of the paravertebral muscles in the lower back and/or the neck. With William A. the retraction was in the lower back.

My work with William progressed in much the same way as with Bryan, who had a similar lower-back syndrome. As the muscles along his lower spine relaxed and extended, William's posture became straighter, and he stood noticeably taller, at least by three quarters of an inch. Soon he was comfortable again. He recognized that he was coming to feel better than he had for a number of years, and so he asked for help to continue developing his sensorimotor capacities. During the sessions that followed, I was warmed to see a nonathlete begin to blossom into a fervent jogger.

When a person has lordosis and a history of lower-back pain, the last thing he should think of doing is running. The vertical shock coming from the ground up through the spine is not absorbed by the bones of the vertebrae, since they are not stacked one upon the other in a near vertical fashion. Instead, the vertical shock is absorbed by the muscles along the lower spine. Put simply, jogging exacerbates the lower-back syndrome, usually bringing on spasms.

Yet, once his lower back was longer and straighter, with the vertebrae stacked up, one on top of the other, William felt that he could do the impossible—at least for him: become a jogger. And he proceeded to do so, building up his running distance daily. Within two months he was doing a daily run from his apartment in San Francisco to the Golden Gate Bridge and back, a total distance of seven miles.

Life is the movement of the body, and the body's sensing of this movement. At the very beginning, the observation was made that living bodies are "individual systems of movement, moving in organized, coordinated, sequential ways." When movement is "organized," "coordinated," and "sequential," it is *timed.* In an absolutely marvelous way, the neural function of timing simultaneously takes every zone of the living body—the face and back, the head and tail, and both sides—and efficiently integrates them into a unified, adroitly adjusted sequence of movements, all designed to perform purposeful tasks, such as playing a vibraphone, plucking a bass, reaching for a glass of water, kicking a ball, or touching the hand of a friend.

The marvelous feature of timing is that it embraces the whole of the available soma. Our own consciousness is not so watchful; it is always switching about, focusing on this thing and that, never able to take in the wholeness and fullness and spherical completeness of our living being. If the operations of our own organic being were solely dependent upon our consciousness, we would not last a day, nor would we be able to take a single step without falling. Conscious attention is a narrow band of activity; it can turn in any direction, but not all at once.

The function of timing is the fourth dimension of our living being, a superior neural function embracing the three dimensions of spatiality with which our bodies are constituted. Whereas consciousness turns in only *one* direction at a time, the timing function turns in *all* directions at a time. It is this omnidirected awareness that actively integrates, monitors, and mobilizes our entire being. At the neural heart of our being—and of all living beings—is a temporal awareness that synthesizes all movements of the body's structure. It is the central cohesiveness that holds our being together as a single process. Without it, we would not be; we would fall asunder into muscular randomness and sensory disorder, not unlike that which is experienced in cerebral palsy or schizophrenia. And we must remember that even as the timing function is the pervasive, all-embracing core of our functional being, so are the central nervous system and the sensorimotor tracts, whose structures are at the living center of this system.

Let us review this. Timing is an essential life function that operates autonomously, involuntarily, and unconsciously, just beneath the restless searchlight of our consciousness. Timing has the function of integrating the whole of our available being into balanced, coordinated, efficient movement and sensation. But the "whole of our available being" is often insufficient to allow us the possibility of balanced, coordinated, efficient movement and sensation. Sometimes our beings are in a habitual state of retraction or fixation or lateralization. In such instances, the function of timing is rendered ineffective: It does not have all that it needs to work with. And thus, our somatic beings are distorted, and our lives diminish in effectiveness.

And this is where consciousness can come to our aid. The unidirectional focus of conscious attention may be a single channel, but it is a channel that can be turned in any direction that attracts it. Normally, conscious attention is turned outward, searching and monitoring the external world, but if we wish it to, we can also direct our awareness inward, searching and monitoring our inner world. When we lift our right foot, we may not be aware of the mobilizing action of our timing function, which is actively balancing the whole of our bodies. If we focus our attention here and there on what is happening in the rest of our bodies, we become aware of what is taking place, and this single-focusing band of awareness can be integrated with the universally focused function of timing. When these two functions meet, a change may occur: By this sensorimotor action, more of the soma can become available for efficient mobilization of our actions.

As already mentioned, when we focus our attention on a tree, it does not affect the tree; but when we focus our attention inwardly upon ourselves and certain movements of our bodies, we affect ourselves. The lives and the bodies of all the persons described in the case histories were inefficient and functionally distorted. The integrative ability of their timing function was limited by what it had to work with. But, with each of them, when their attention was directed inward and they were taught to focus their sensory awareness on formerly unconscious movements in their bodies, their bodies and the efficiency of their lives were transformed. When sensory awareness is directed inward, at movements that are atrophied or unlearned, it can liberate and reclaim these unmoving and forgotten aspects of our living being, making them available to us for a more efficient and fulfilling life.

All living creatures possess this function of timing, whose purpose it is to integrate the three dimensions of somatic being into effective actions. Only one creature, the human being, possesses a sensory awareness that can be directed away from the external world and focused inwardly on the internal functioning of our somatic process. When this sensory awareness is directed inward to the undeveloped or atrophied processes of our living bodies, these processes change—and they change for the better, because more has been integrated into the ongoing process of our lives. In brief, we become more adaptable by integrating new fragments into the whole process of our central nervous system. The total somatic process is thereby improved: Our actions improve, our balance improves, our thinking improves, our judgment improves, our emotional tone improves—in short, our lives improve. These improvements occur because, like a spade turning up new earth, the focusing of awareness on requisite movement patterns frees more of our somatic being for integration by the primordial function of timing.

Standing, facing, handling, and timing—these are the four dimensions that lie at the heart of all somas and that lie at the heart of human beings, just beneath the restless focus of their consciousness. The first three dimensions constitute the spatiality of the living body, its substance and its shape. The fourth dimension constitutes the temporality of the living body, integrating the three lower functions into an efficient, adaptive process. Taken together, these four dimensions constitute the ancient, somatic heart of all living creatures. They are the "old soma," the archesoma that is the functioning core of all things living, no matter what may be their species difference.

Commentary: The Function of Timing

When we reflect upon the way in which we function, we must not lose the historical, somatic viewpoint, which offers us a steady grasp on what is central to understanding ourselves versus what is peripheral to this understanding. What is central to any clear understanding of ourselves, and all of life, is that *all somatic functions are movements.* The different functions of each species are the characteristic intentional actions of each species. In the nonhuman species, these intentional actions are genetically "fixed," as the ethologists express it; in the human species, however, intentional actions are unfixed. They are, instead, learned through communication with other human beings.

Human somatology begins with a forgetting of the delusionary words *mind* and *body* and their replacement with the working terms *function* and *structure.* Whatever is meant by *body* is far more adequately suggested when we speak of physiological, organic structure. This is because the word *function* has to do with movement, and movement is the essential characteristic of life and the living process.

The functions of standing, facing, handling, and timing

are primordial and constitutive in the sense that when and if life is discovered in other solar systems, we can be certain that it will also be constituted by these same primordial functions. They have predictive value.

The somatic viewpoint teaches us that the most important functions in human beings are functions that are not specifically human. Whatever the specific ways in which any species lives and survives in the environment, there is an underlying core of functions upon which these specific actions are based. In order for there to be a soma that can adapt to the environment, there must be a core of somatic functions that makes environmental adaptation possible.

In order for a creature to function well in this world, its primordial core of somatic functions must be in good order. These functions are in good order when each of them retains its "bias," that is, when each of the four functions has the nonhomeostatic imbalance that characterizes life functions. We know, for example, that a balance of the vertical plane would be a directionality that is equally downward and upward: That would be homeostasis of the vertical plane. But the primordial functions are not so constituted. The first function has a predilection, a bias for moving upward; if it does not do so, it is malfunctioning.

If we are to understand how we, or any other living creature, can best survive and succeed in this world, we must look to the positive biases that are built into each primordial somatic function. The soma prefers to stand up, rather than slump downward. The soma prefers to face forward, rather than turn backward. The soma prefers to handle what it aims for, rather than miss the mark. The soma prefers to time its movements in efficiently coordinated sequences, rather than remain in spatial rigidity.

These four biases are essential to the constitution of the soma and are essential to its well-being; if they become merely balanced or underbalanced, they automatically lower the efficiency of the soma and threaten its viability in the world. The effectiveness of the life of any human being rests, first of all, on the proper operation of these four biased functions. If one or more are malfunctioning, the general adaptive behavior of the human being becomes distorted.

It is the ability to time itself efficiently that is the grand accomplishment of life's body, and it is the timing function that gives life its general characteristic of integrated movement and process. Life's timing process is somewhat like a juggling act, in which elements are kept in motion in a series. It is a continuing process that is always incomplete, by definition. At any given instant in the soma's process—its movement, metabolism, and directionality—something is "in the air" and has not yet come down. At any given instant, the soma is in a state of incompleteness and suspense: It is waiting for an event that has not yet happened. This is to say that *the stratagem of somatic process is to organize movement via temporal sequence* so as to reduce entropy and gain energy.

It is the contrivance of life to invest in the future, namely, to risk an expenditure of energy that is not instantly recuperable but comes about only after a delay. It is life's design to keep its process moving during this delay in recuperation and rebalancing by reinvesting itself in new ventures.

What must be stressed is that this investment in the

future is a deliberate risk on the part of the soma; it is the deliberate provocation of an event in expectation of rewarding consequences. The soma risks because it is confident of the gain.

That is the word: *confidence.* The deliberate risks ceaselessly ventured by living beings are done in absolute confidence of reward. The reward is not merely awaited, it is expected. And what is expected by this process is *a surplus of energy,* generated by the higher efficiency of the timing process.

In summary, life is movement, and the sequential process of life is the timed coordination of its movements. This process risks incompleteness with absolute confidence of future completeness, and because of this confidence, it projects yet further sequences of actions. This is the unstable-yet-stable nature of somatic process.

Now that we have a more refined view of the timing process, we can appreciate how this confident risking of futurity teaches us something about life that has not yet been firmly established in biology. Hitherto, biologists have followed the Darwinian theory of evolution in the minimal sense of asserting that the basic rule of life is to survive. This homeostatic, hold-your-own estimate of life's fundamental drive betrays the degree to which biology has not yet transcended the static, spatialized thinking of the physical sciences. Merely to survive is not simply a minimal description of the project of life; it is an insufficient description.

Everything we know about living creatures tells us that the soma was not made to hold its own and survive but *to do more than that: to expand and grow and evolve.* That is precisely what somas have done during their astonishingly prolific pilgrimage of 3,400,000,000 years, and to fail to see this fact is to fail to see the genius of organic beings.

The confident risk taking of the soma is not the action of a survivor, it is the action of an expander and grower, who, through the efficiency of its process, has an excess of energy. The least worry of the soma is homeostasis and survival—that is assumed, otherwise the soma would not ceaselessly risk imbalance and insecurity. The soma, from its origins, went beyond the minimal need for stability and, as a higher-order synthesis, used its surplus of energy for diversification, expansion, and growth. Mutation and the evolution of new species were foredestined for such a creature.

Contrary to traditional biological thinking, *growth is open-ended; it is a venture of risk.* Growth is not a static, repeated cycle, nor has it ever been. It is always expansion toward more than what has been. Only conceptions are static. Life grows, expands, evolves toward an open-ended future of its own contrivance. Some human beings may hang on to life, just managing to survive, but all somas prior to human somas have confidently expanded their number and their variety into the universe, almost as if the universe existed only for the purpose of supporting and lending itself to the project of life's expansion.

For life to be, it had to discover, mutation by mutation, ways of standing and balancing against the gravity of the world. This may sound remote from anything human, until we reflect that the earliest genetically given reflexes of human infants have to do with balance and upright orientation with gravity. The function of standing upright in balance is so basic that anything disturbing the development of that function will prevent the development of normal "human" intelligence.

For life to be a part of this world, it had to express the second spatial dimension of depth, and it did so by developing a face, in the middle of which was a mouth that always headed into the world. Facing and heading into the world are the ways in which somas move toward what they need. Human beings who do not learn to face and move toward what they want do not obtain what they need to survive, either emotionally or physiologically. Facing is a positive and optimistic function of directing oneself toward the satisfaction of one's appetite. The human being who is unable to look directly at what he wants is a person who is crippled with dissatisfaction and unfulfilled needs.

Just as unavoidably, the third spatial dimension of width imposed laterality and symmetry upon the body of life. Somas have two sides. When one side is used to *seize* the world, the other side coordinates with it. Human beings have evolved from their ambidextrous ancestry as, essentially, right-handed beings. They have specialized, and this specialization is reflected in the functions of the central nervous system. All human beings must learn either right-sided or left-sided specialization in order to reach for and grasp what they want; otherwise, they are unable to handle the world with enough efficiency to guarantee their survival and growth. In addition, we have hardly touched upon the momentous fact that mankind's unique ability to use language is inextricably bound up with handedness.

It is timing that brings the three somatic dimensions together as an integrated neural process. It is this function that gives integrity and wholeness to the soma. In prehuman somas, we have noticed the astounding abilities that living creatures have in coordinating certain actions crucial to their survival. Ethologists call these abilities fixed action patterns, and they are genetically passed on from generation to generation as forms of preadapted "learning"—whether it be the migrations of birds or the stalking habits of dogs. In human beings, however, the timing function undergoes an extraordinary mutation. It loses the guiding control of inherited fixed action patterns and comes under the guiding control of something distinctively human: learning. What is learned by the timing function is not simply the ability to coordinate a sequence of three-dimensional movements but rather the ability to coordinate them toward an efficient fulfillment of the soma's wants.

The significance of this is that somas are not merely in balance with the physical world; they are not only in homeostasis with the environment. Instead, somas are always risking imbalance and instability in order to move toward some accomplishment. It is a biological law that all somatic functions have a purpose, otherwise they would never have evolved and survived. This means that *the body of life is goal oriented; it is telenomic.* The great Nobel laureate Jacques Monod laid absolute stress on this in his *Chance and Necessity.* As he sees it, "one of the fundamental characteristics common to all living beings without exception is that of being *objects endowed with a purpose or project,* which at the same time they exhibit in their structure and carry out through their performances." This biological intentionality "is essential to the very definition of living beings" (Monod, 1972, p. 9).

The four somatic functions that dwell within us have their own ancient and wise intentions, and it behooves us to learn to understand these basic purposes that operate quietly in our somatic core. These four functions constitute the archesoma that knows what it needs and wants; and, in the profoundest biological sense, this is also what each of *us* needs and wants. It is a question of becoming aware of this marvelous living core and of understanding its transparent wisdom. And, thanks to the integrative function of timing, this wisdom is the wisdom of efficiency, comfort, and ease.

TWO / SOMATIC EDUCATION

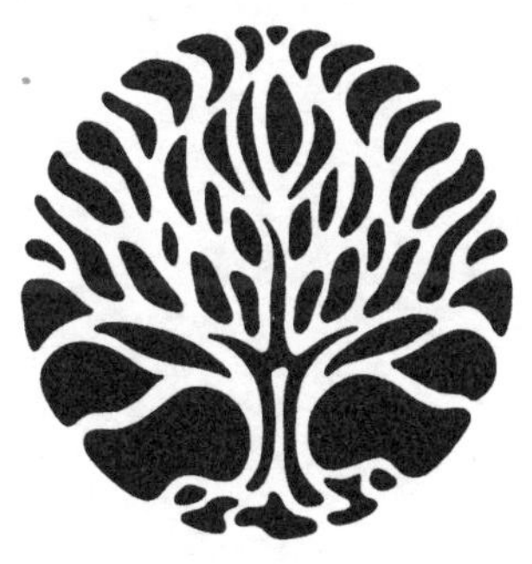

1 / the nature of learning

The entire brain of an adult male weighs something in the neighborhood of fifty ounces—or about fourteen hundred grams. The brain is a colossal organ. It is an aggregate of some twelve billion neurons, most of which (nine billion) are concentrated in the top layer, the cerebral cortex. In the center of these nerve cells, like the main pole of a tent upon which all else hangs, stands the sensorimotor system.

This massive assemblage of nerve cells is united in performing one dual function: moving the body in coordination and integrating the sensory information that it receives from the body. The neurophysiologist Roger W. Sperry has concluded that the sole product of brain function is muscular coordination. He has even refined this judgment by saying that the entire output of our thinking mechanism goes into the motor system. This is to say that when we think, we are either activating muscles or, at the very least, activating motor neurons. When one realizes that this judgment is generally supported by the consensus of brain research during the past few decades, it becomes obvious that the ancient conception of human beings having a mind that thinks and a separate body that acts is fairly well debunked. The human being is a single being, a soma, that is self-moving, self-sensing, and self-integrating.

Because of its preeminent position in the central nervous system, both functionally and structurally, the sensorimotor system deserves a closer inspection. The most obvious structural feature of this system is that it is in the center of the body, built into the entire length of the spine all the way up to the top center of the cerebral cortex, with the motor nerves placed just to the front of center and the sensory nerves just to the rear (figures 1 and 2). Just as obvious is the fact that the sensorimotor tracts in the

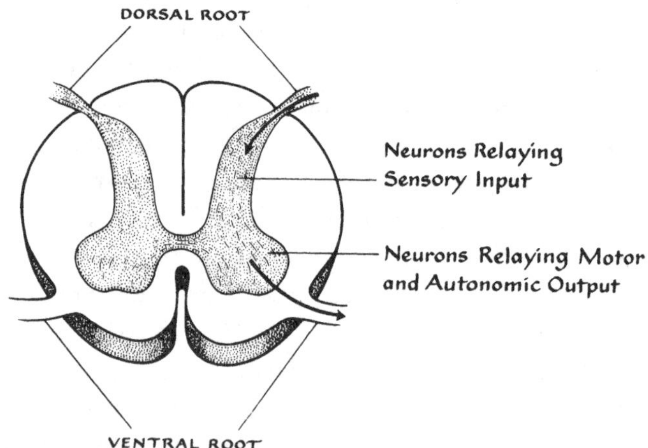

Figure 1. *Sensory and Motor Tracts in the Spinal Cord*

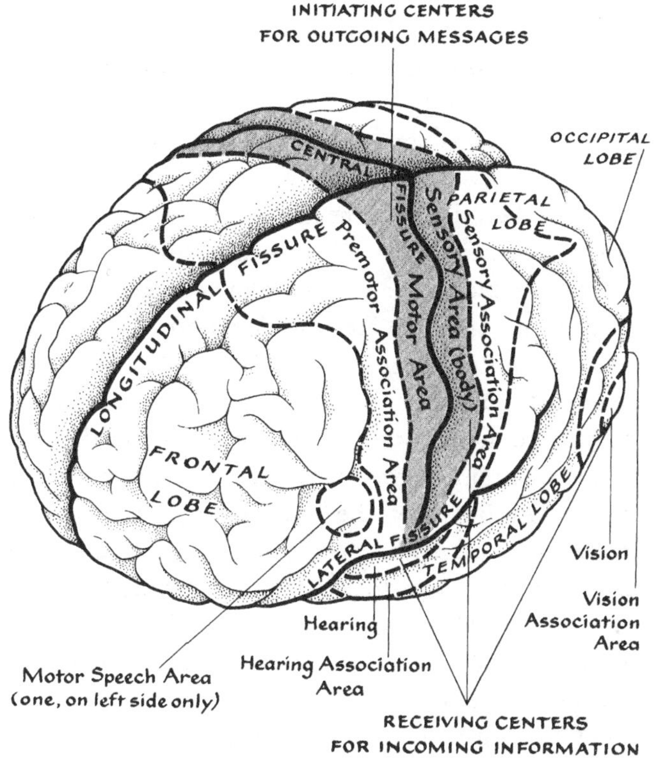

Figure 2. *Sensory and Motor Tracts in the Cerebral Cortex*

brain's left side cross over to control these functions on the right side of the body, with the tracts in the right hemisphere controlling those on the left side of the body. This crossover phenomenon indicates the integral way in which the nervous system controls the body. Offhand one might wonder why the left brain does not control the left side of the body and the right brain the right side—like two identical halves stuck together. But neither the brain nor the body are two halves united; rather, they are a single somatic unit, bifurcated into two working components. The crossover of neural circuits is the structural sign of the soma's unity.

There is a less obvious feature of the sensorimotor system that has, only gradually, been mapped out: This is the way in which the neurons in these tracts are arranged. It is a most rational arrangement, as orderly in its layout as are the ascending keys on a piano keyboard. In fact, it is quite similar. Just as pressing down on the white key of middle C activates the striking of the C string in the piano, so does stimulation of a neuron in these tracts activate the corresponding muscle cell or sensory cell in the body.

During brain surgery, when the skull has been opened at the top, just over the sensorimotor tracts, neurosurgeons have stimulated these neurons with a tiny filament charged with a very small amount of electricity, measured in millivolts. When the filament touched the neurons leading to the muscles of the foot or cheek or thumb, those particular muscles would contract. When the same filament was brushed across the neurons in the sensory tract corresponding to the foot or cheek or thumb, and so forth, that person—who, surprisingly, could be kept comfortably awake during the procedure—would report feeling a sensation not in the brain but in the foot or cheek or thumb, respectively, just as if one were plunking different keys of the piano and activating different notes.

But the similarity of the sensorimotor system to the rational arrangement of a piano goes much further than this. The orderly layout of the neurons in these tracts sketches out, as it were, a picture of the entire human body from bottom to top.

Figures 3 and 4 show how the arrangement of nerve cells in the sensory and motor tracts of the cortex represents the human body from bottom to top. It is as if a little man were sketched out along these tracts, and for this reason it has come to be called the sensory homunculus and the motor homunculus. The feet of the homunculus begin at the longitudinal fissure, which separates the two hemispheres of the brain. Then the neuronal picture of the body sketches its way up through the leg, hip, trunk, shoulder, arm, and hand as we trace the tracts from the longitudinal fissure out to the side of the brain. Further on, the neurons for the face, lips, tongue, and vocal organs are sketched out. If we were to run a lightly charged filament across this neuronal keyboard, the muscles and senses would be activated in a rational, sequential manner. There would be a rising contraction of the muscles and an ascending arpeggio of sensations.

Upon looking closer at the little man, we begin to notice some unusual features of this neural body. The first and perhaps most obvious feature is the enormous space allotted to the hands and face and the small amount allotted to the legs and trunk of the body. Although the legs and trunk are a major portion of the bodily structure, they are a minor portion of the neural structure—a fact that puts us in a better position to judge which bodily functions are the most significant from a neural point of view. In viewing the homunculus, we are, to a large extent, viewing the functional human being as contrasted with the structural human being; in a rather exact sense, we are getting nearer to what the living human body is like: the human soma.

The homunculus shows us that the greatest investment

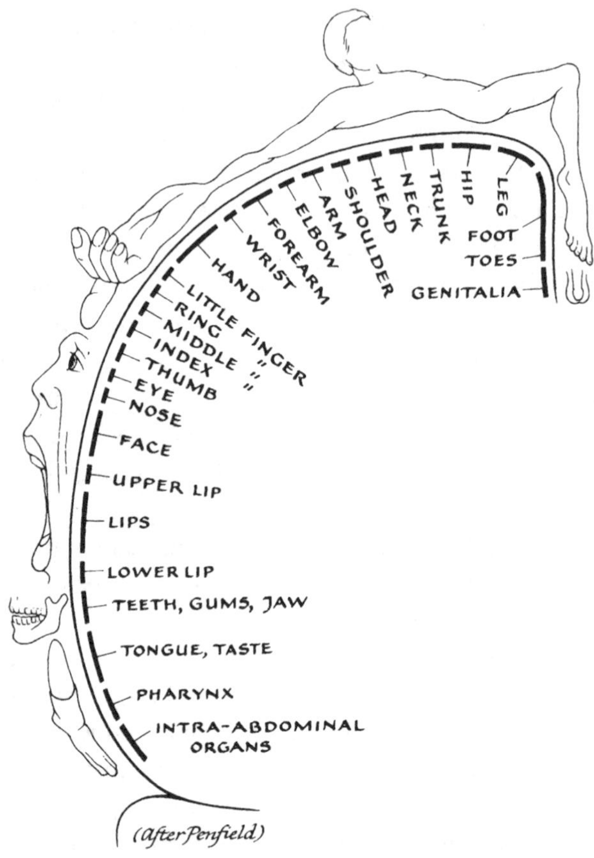

Figure 3. *The Sensory Cortex Homunculus*

of neuronal space is in the hands and face. This is instructive. Inasmuch as the brain structure that we are viewing has successfully evolved over millions of years, the homunculus lets us know that having a hand with fingers and a face with a mouth is central to our survival. To live, we must eat, and to eat we must manage to find food, grasp it, and bring it to our mouth. But we not only use our mouth to eat, we use it to speak, and so the lips and tongue

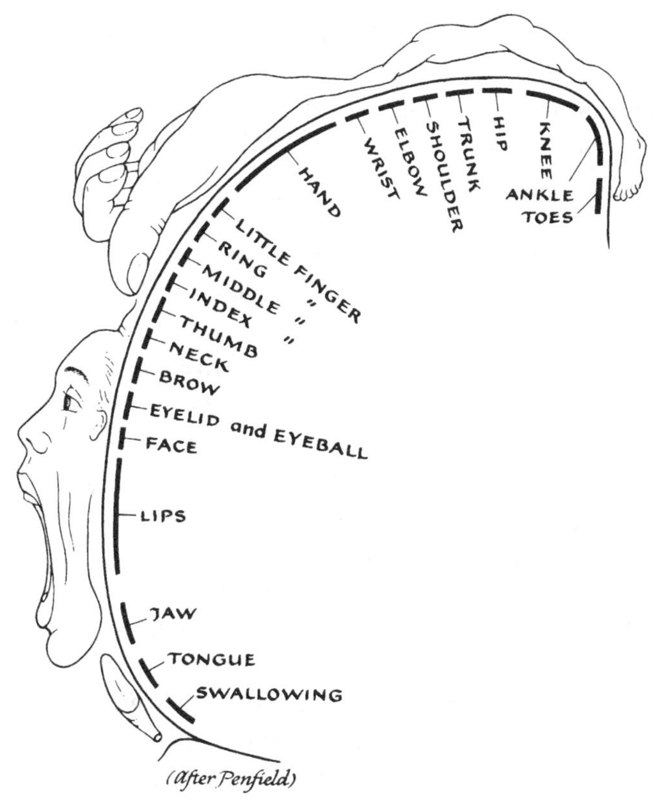

Figure 4. *The Motor Cortex Homunculus*

and throat have a rich and complex neuronal supply for the subtleties of speech, even as the fingers have a rich supply for the subtleties of handling and manipulating. The homunculus instructs us that human beings do not simply function as mouths that forage for themselves; we are also language users, who communicate, and tool makers, who construct.

Another striking feature of the neuronal arrangement

of these sensorimotor tracts is the separation of the face from the rest of the body. The body of the homunculus extends from its toes up to its shoulders, neck, and head, but there is no face. It has its own special functions that distinguish it, neurally, from the side of the body. What we see, then, is the laterality of the neural body—the prime feature of each side being the hand—and the faciality of the neural body—the prime feature being the mouth. The homunculus shows a dominant commitment to two main functional areas: the lateral functions of handling and the frontal functions of facing. This neural disjunction between lateral functions and frontal functions is further emphasized by the curious fact that the facing functions are inverted in relation to the handling functions. Whereas the body's side is curved over, upside down, the facial area is right side up. This distinctive position of the face should remind us that the face contains not only a mouth for eating and speaking but also the senses of vision, hearing, and smell that give information to the rest of the body about what is out in front of it and about which way it is to go. The homuncular arrangement suggests to us that the face has the distinct function of guiding and leading the body forward so that it might reach out and handle what the homunculus wants.

The sensorimotor homunculus is a creature made for perception and action. It is designed for the process of sensate movement. But what we see is not the whole sensorimotor system, merely its highly instructive cortical surface. The neurons of these tracts descend down to other integrative centers that lie just beneath the layer of the cortex and that relate the functions of these tracts to the sensory association area and the premotor association area, as well as to the occipital lobe, which controls vision, and the temporal lobe, where hearing is processed. This you will see in figure 2. What you will not see, however, are the three semicircular canals of the vestibular system, which is lodged in the bony substance of the mastoid section of the skull. These three fluid-filled canals are directly linked to central integrative areas of the brain and cerebellum. They pass information to the soma's face and two sides about where the vertical up-down line of gravity is. The vestibular system is the sanctuary of the standing function.

Another thing you will not see is the timing function, not only because functions are not observable except through the ways they move structure but also because the timing function is not anywhere; rather, it is everywhere. The timing function is the integrative function of the living body. As such, it is all pervasive and everywhere, otherwise it could not coordinate and synthesize the combined sensory and motor process of the entire soma. The timing function is a supreme integrative function of the central nervous system, yet it has no specific organ. It pervades all organs with its hegemony.

Even though we have not caught a glimpse of the timing function, we have seen its lair. We have seen the neural keyboard upon which it plays. Better still, we have gained an appreciation of how the structure and functions of the living body intermesh in an indissoluble unity. We can, perhaps, better understand Roger Sperry's judgment that "the entire output of our thinking mechanism goes into the motor system."

The implication is that thinking is a physical act. More specifically, it means that thinking is a motor act, triggering the motor neurons in the motor cortex, which directly connect with the muscles of the body. What Sperry is suggesting is a somatic viewpoint, namely, that thinking is movement—actual physical movement of the living body. Several thousand years of philosophical and religious belief may well cause us to bridle at this implication, but it could well be that these millennia of metaphysical and theological beliefs have kept us from an authentic understanding of ourselves as living human beings. Just as Dante was able to discover Heaven only by descending through the bottom door of Hell, so we may be able to discover the authentic sources of spiritual belief only by venturing more deeply into the somatic inwardness of ourselves.

One of the scientific pioneers in the investigation of the relationship between thinking and motor activity was Edmund Jacobson. His research eventually led him to develop a famous clinical procedure called progressive relaxation, which is useful in reducing states of high tension and anxiety. Beginning in 1927, Jacobson built an electrical apparatus to record muscular tension and, over the years, showed conclusively that there is a close and indisputable relationship between thinking and muscle tension. When subjects were asked to engage in abstract thinking, he found that speech muscles were prominently activated. He also found that all mental activity decreased to the degree that muscle tension decreased (Jacobson, 1938, 1970).

Along this same line, Smith, Brown, Toman, and Goodman (1947) performed an experiment to find out what would happen to the thinking process if all muscles were paralyzed. This was done by administering a curare-type drug to a volunteer subject; when total paralysis occurred, artificial respiration was given to the subject, because the diaphragm had ceased to move the pulmonary cavity. During the time of the experiment there was no lapse of consciousness, but the subject reported that he was ineffective in focusing on anything. This is a deficit in sensorimotor functioning, in particular of the facing and handling functions.

Another pioneer in this field was Roland C. Davis (1939), who discovered that when subjects were asked to think out a problem in multiplication, the muscles of the dominant hand began to move as if the subject were writing.

One of the most curious discoveries about the relationship between thought and motor activity is that reported by F. J. McGuigan (1970) with a person who had auditory hallucinations. McGuigan placed electrodes around the speech muscles of the subject and asked him to indicate when he began hallucinating the voice. At the moment when he indicated that the voice was speaking, McGuigan noticed that there was a slight, continuing movement in the speech muscles. The subject was speaking to himself without being aware of it; that is, it requires motor activity to hallucinate a voice.

Perhaps the most extensive research on the relation of motor activity to mental functions is that carried out for thirty years at McGill University by Robert Malmo. One of the intriguing areas of Malmo's work is his research on EMG gradients, which is the rise or fall (gradients) of muscle tension recorded by an electromyograph (EMG). The importance of this research is that it shows not simply the relationship between thinking and muscle tension but how muscle tension changes when thoughts go from pleasant to unpleasant topics. For example, persons with chronic headaches or neck pains allowed EMG electrodes to be placed on the muscles of the area that had pain. Then, during the interview, if the topics were unpleasant or if distracting noises came into the room, the subject's muscle tension would begin rising; at the point of its zenith, the subject would complain of the familiar headache or pain in the neck. The considerable work done by Malmo in this area has definitely made it clear that in the course of entertaining emotion-laden topics, all human beings unconsciously undergo ascents or descents in muscular tension.

One study along this line was performed in Malmo's laboratory by Wallerstein (1954). He had subjects lying in bed listening to a good detective story from a tape recorder while muscle activity was recorded from EMGs on the forehead muscle. What Wallerstein discovered was that as the subject's interest in the story grew, so did the muscle gradient in the forehead. As the story moved to its climax, so did the gradient move to its highest tension. But then, as soon as the story was finished, the EMG gradient dropped back down to what it was before. Wallerstein had shown the somatic fact that the internal, proprioceptive experience of growing interest and suspense involves the experience of gradually contracting muscles. When the suspense is over, the muscle tension is over.

An unusual and disturbing fact was turned up in the course of these experiments. If the story was interrupted and not completed, the muscular tension remained—there was "residual tension." What emerged was this: When human beings are engaged in a goal-oriented activity, the EMG gradient of certain muscles will rise steadily to the point of attaining that goal; then when the job is finished, the gradient will drop. If, however, the work is not completed, the residual tension continues in the muscles, dropping down only very slowly.

The McGill University lab did another experiment on this phenomenon. Two groups of subjects were asked to tell a story about a picture they were shown; these subjects had EMG monitors to record their speech-muscle tension. After listening to their stories, a psychiatrist responded by praising half of the subjects, whereas he criticized the other half. Those who were praised for their good performance all showed a sharp drop in their muscle tension. However, those who were criticized for their bad performance lost none of the tension they had built up. The residual tension remained, not only in the subjects but also in the psychiatrist doing the criticizing, for he, too, had EMG monitors! It is of some interest to add that the subjects' residual tension could be removed, but only when *another* member of the staff explained what had been happening and reassured the subjects of their competence.

These laboratory findings have immediate bearing on our understanding of how functionally caused ailments come about. We are, of course, referring to situations of stress, and stress is a word that the celebrated Hans Selye has, through his own extensive research, brought into full medical recognition. Stress is a demand made upon the living body when one is in the course of goal-oriented activity. What the research at McGill University and elsewhere has shown us is that expectation and suspense are not "mental" states; they are somatic states. All of our being is affected. And, by the same token, disappointment, delayed satisfaction, and failure are not simply "mental" difficulties; they are somatic difficulties.

If rising muscle gradients accompany all goal-oriented behavior, and if delayed satisfaction or continual incompletion maintains this muscle tension, then we have a way of understanding how somatic distortion occurs. The high-pressure jobs of Pat and Charlie are carrot-before-the-horse jobs where goal-orientation is constant and where the completion of one goal is submerged in the fact that there are simultaneously ten other goals not yet achieved and some others that have failed to be achieved. Pat and Charlie and all of the other persons we have described lived daily lives that did everything to increase the muscular tension of their bodies and nothing to bring it down. The weekends and the martinis were not enough to erase this large residual tension, and when Monday came, they were up at six o'clock chasing more goals and more carrots until the time came that they were ready to collapse. They were so distorted, somatically, that they could no longer function efficiently.

Contemporary culture is destructive in the way it invites people to accept situations—the duties of the working husband or those of the urban wife and mother—that are attritional. Given enough time in these situations, human beings are gradually distorted beyond endurance. The muscular tension builds up, hindering the easy movements of their bodies, and the sensations of this tension feed back to their awareness, deluging their consciousness with the nonverbal siren of anxiety and pain.

What the neurophysiological research of the past several decades tells us is that the kind of thoughts we think determines the quality and effectiveness of our lives. Because thinking is an action of the entire body that mobilizes the entire sensorimotor system, the nature of our thinking activity automatically determines the nature of our bodily activity. If we turn the same anxious thoughts over in our minds day after day, then it is certain that we are tensing and activating certain contractions in our bodies day after day. And it is just as certain that these afflicted parts of our bodies will, through this daily abuse, become fatigued and damaged.

When we think the same thoughts of revenge over and over again, we are activating the muscles and glands of our bodies over and over again. When we repeat the same thought of disappointment over and over, we are repeatedly stamping its motor power into the tissues of our body until they sag in forlornness. When we repeatedly think thoughts or memories of hurt, despair, anger, or fear, we are physically injuring ourselves; we are engaging in self-destruction.

You can be sure that the weight of neurophysiological evidence is massively on the side of those who advise us to think positive thoughts rather than negative thoughts—if it is possible. But given the demands placed upon us, many persons are rarely in a situation where they can entertain positive thoughts. Contemporary culture is, for most citizens, an oppressive pall that hovers over them throughout their lives. The simple task of maintaining economic and social status is more anxiety filled than it was even half a century ago. If, in addition to a person's job, he has the daily experience of reading the newspaper and the nightly experience of watching the evening newscast, he has enough disappointment and apprehension and foreboding to guarantee that the residual muscular tension in his body will not drop a whit.

There is no easy solution to this problem. There certainly is no permanent solution. But the first step is to look at the problem and understand it. A somatic understanding of ourselves allows us to understand, to a large degree, what is happening to us and why our thoughts, our culture, and our individual ways of living affect us in the thoroughly physiological and emotional ways that they do. By understanding ourselves and the fuller aspects of our functioning, we are empowered to help ourselves. We may be able to do nothing about our culture and, perhaps, little about our job, but we can do much about ourselves and the way we process our experience.

This discussion of somatic distortion and of the neurophysiological research that is relevant to the causes of this distortion has made one thing clear: Our total beings can be transformed by our daily experience and by what we focus our consciousness on. So far, this discussion has dealt with only the negative and distorting transformations that can occur to us. But we know that our sensorimotor systems are just as capable of positive and life-giving transformations. Quite apart from society and culture, we can redeem ourselves and take control of our sensorimotor growth, just as easily as we can abandon ourselves and lose control. We simply need to know how, so that we can chart our way through the maze. It is a question of learning—learning those patterns that are easier and more efficient and unlearning the patterns that are painful and inefficient.

2 / the somatic educators

THE GENTLE PIONEERS

Matthias Alexander and Elsa Gindler

The two earliest pioneers in somatic education confirmed the adage that necessity is the mother of invention. F. Matthias Alexander and Elsa Gindler made their discoveries in the somatic realm because they had no other option.

If he was to continue his stage career, Alexander had no other option than to find a way to improve his voice. He was a Shakespearean actor in Sydney, Australia, during the close of the last century. Increasingly, he was plagued by a loss of voice, which he believed was caused not by a weak constitution but, rather, by *misuse* of his voice. Speech clinics were unknown at the time, and Alexander decided to study himself and diagnose what was wrong.

To this end, he used the simplest form of biofeedback device, a mirror. He stood before it, began reciting his lines, and watched his movements. Like all things somatic, at first it was too obvious to notice; then, eventually, he began to isolate one particular movement of his head and neck that he constantly made while orating. He would curve his neck so that his chin went up and the back of his head sank downward, as if dropping into the chest. It was a somewhat cringing movement, typical enough in many persons, but Alexander saw that it was a distortion of his throat passage, causing him to strain his vocal chords. This observation of the typical, but unconscious, movements of somatic retraction was the beginning of the Alexander Technique.

In 1904 Alexander came to London and, during the course of the next forty years, became renowned for his success in teaching others how to change the habitual posture of their neck, shoulders, and back. The changes in people's bodies were so surprising and extraordinary that George Bernard Shaw sapiently concluded that the Alexander Technique was "the beginning of a far-reaching science." John Dewey attributed his long and robustly creative life to Alexander's work and proclaimed it "the new direction that is needed in all education." Later, Aldous Huxley was to say, "Alexander's technique gives us the things we have been looking for . . . a method for the creative conscious control of the whole psycho-physical organism." The great ethologist Niko Tinbergen praised the Alexander Technique in his acceptance speech for the Nobel prize in medicine in 1973.

The public recognition of his technique was such that Alexander began teaching and certifying others to do his work. These teachers spread from Great Britain throughout the British Commonwealth and into the United States, instructing those with postural disorders how to inhibit and overcome their imbalances. They taught others by showing them how to use their bodies more efficiently and comfortably. They used their hands, holding the learner's head and chin in a certain position while he practiced sitting up from a supine position. This is a direct manner of showing a person what it feels like to use his body in a different way. Not only does the teacher hold the head or shoulders or back in a new position, but as the pupil practices, the teacher verbally reinforces what it feels like by saying such things as, "Neck free, head forward and up, back lengthen and widen."

The significant thing about the Alexander Technique is that it works. It works because it invites the learner to become aware of the misuse of his body and to inhibit this habitual way of moving; simultaneously, it makes the learner aware of a more efficient use of his body, gives him a verbal command to reinforce it, and asks him to practice inhibiting the old and reinforcing the new movement patterns throughout the normal working day—while typing, washing dishes, reading, or working with tools. Gradually the person's posture changes; he stands taller, more balanced, and he moves more easily and gracefully, "grace" being the expression of an effortless efficiency.

Perhaps the central discovery of Alexander was that the head-neck region was the area of "primary control" of the human body. The head contains the organs of balance and of distance perception. It guides and triggers the responses of the rest of the body. If something is wrong in the balance and movement of the head, then the rest of the body will be in an unbalanced strain. By the same token, if one wishes to change the general posture of the body, one must start with the head-neck region.

Elsa Gindler was a Berlin physical educator, and her

work developed out of the fact that she was tubercular and poor. As a young woman during the early part of the century, she was distressed to learn that she was consumptive. The physician urged a prolonged convalescence in Switzerland during which the lung most affected could be healed. Unable to afford such a luxury, she determined to gain such control over her breathing that she would use only one lung, allowing the other to rest. She did this by observing her internal sensations, differentiating the movements of her throat, rib cage, diaphragm, and stomach until she could both sense and control each lung in breathing. By this simple and startlingly direct method the infected lung was restored to normal function—a fact that her physician refused to accept, preferring to believe that miracles sometimes happen.

But Gindler knew it was no miracle; it was the result of being searchingly attentive to what was taking place within her body. Her self-imposed task of learning to rest one lung resulted in more than her own cure: It resulted in her discovery that *the more human beings are aware of their internal sensations, the better they can function.*

She recognized that human awareness offers a direct way of changing and improving the functions of the body. Because it was a human ability that was the agent for change, she called her subsequent work *Arbeit am Menschen* (Work on People). Gindler had discovered that human awareness is not a "psychological," "mental," or "spiritual" function; it is an actual physiological function. Although she did not use the term, she saw human awareness as a somatic function.

Elsa Gindler took seriously a phenomenon with which human beings have always been familiar: that directing one's attention to some part of one's body is an action that immediately affects that bodily part. If, at this instant, you continue to hold this book exactly as you are doing, without changing it, and you notice the relative tension or comfort of your hands and fingers, it is like turning a spotlight on your hands. Whatever sensations you were feeling a moment ago in your hands are minor compared with what you feel now. Your awareness highlights what is actually happening in your hands, and if your hands were unconsciously overtensed or uncomfortably positioned, you may notice that you now automatically adjust your hands so that they hold the book more easily.

Sensory awareness of the inner kinesthetic and proprioceptive feedback of our neural system predisposes the muscular system to adjust itself to more efficient functioning. This is not "mind over matter"; rather, it shows how one somatic function is linked with another, that is, how the sensory system is intimately linked with the muscular system.

We have seen how, in the sensorimotor homunculus, one somatic function is linked with another. And when sensory awareness of the state of one's muscles results in the adjustment of those muscles, it is a case not of "mind over matter" but of sensory over motor. However, the changed motor patterns cycle back and give new sensory impressions, which again readjust the muscular coordination, and so on. It is a constant feedback loop that never ceases, from birth until death.

So if Elsa Gindler discovered that greater sensory awareness leads to more efficient muscular control, she was recognizing the importance of certain neurophysiological facts that no one had thought to take advantage of.

She believed that human beings were capable of a degree of self-correction and self-transformation not possible in any other living species.

And if Matthias Alexander discovered that a person's physical posture could be radically modified by directing his awareness to a specific way of "using" (i.e., moving) himself, then we know he was doing the same thing as Gindler. Neither of them, however, made these discoveries through their knowledge of neurophysiology. They made their discoveries within themselves as immediately verifiable facts.

Not only have Alexander's students spread throughout the world, Elsa Gindler's have as well. In her Berlin studios Gindler trained numerous practitioners of her gentle art of awareness. One of them, Charlotte Selver, brought these insights to the United States, and over the course of several decades Selver's teaching profoundly influenced the thought of Erich Fromm, the development of Fritz Perls' Gestalt psychology, and the attitude of Wilhelm Reich toward breathing.

But one of the most interesting effects of Selver's work, which she calls Sensory Awareness, was the response of the Anglo-American philosopher Alan Watts. Upon first becoming acquainted with Selver's Sensory Awareness, Watts exclaimed, "Why, this is the living Zen!" Selver, at that time, knew nothing of Zen Buddhism and wondered how the work of a Berlin physical educator could have anything to do with the practice of a Japanese sect. Eventually, however, she saw the undeniable similarities between the practices of Sensory Awareness and those of Zen Buddhism.

Both the nature of Zen Buddhism and its practice are

clarified and demystified when we realize that it is a system of somatic education. Zen practitioners have firmly insisted that Zen is not a religion, that it deals with the reality of things as they are. Yet Westerners were puzzled as to how one could obtain "enlightenment" without a system of doctrine and teaching. It is as if Zen spokesmen such as Daisetz Suzuki were paralleling what Moshe Feldenkrais was later to say about Functional Integration: "The first principle of Zen Buddhism is that there is no principle."

Zen is a practice; it is a "way" and a "how" of living in which total attention, full awareness is the goal. "How can I obtain enlightenment, master?" asks the Zen apprentice. The Zen master replies, "Sit down and shut up." "Is that all?" the apprentice asks. "Yes," says the master. "Be quiet and learn how to sit. When you've done that, come back." These paradoxical aspects of Zen training have always puzzled Westerners, who sought for some slyly hidden metaphysical meaning where there was none. Don't think, don't talk, don't analyze, don't conceptualize is the suggestion; instead, perceive yourself, notice what is happening within, practice awareness. When you are aware of what it means "to sit," when you are aware of what it means "to breathe," then you will move into the serenity, the emotional balance and peacefulness of enlightenment.

The enlightenment sought by the Zen devotee is somatic enlightenment, and it comes with the gradual discovery of efficiency and ease in somatic functioning. It is not a way of thinking or of believing. It is, quite simply, a way of living the philosophical truth of things.

So we should not be surprised that the way of learning Functional Integration, the Alexander Technique, or Sensory Awareness is not dissimilar from the way in which one trains to be a Zen Buddhist. None of these disciplines is designed to help others by imposing a system on them; on the contrary, the intellectual preoccupation with a system is cast aside because, before thought, there is already an anciently ordained and evolved system: the archesoma that dwells at the core of the human animal.

The leading Zen master in the Americas, Richard Baker Roshi, says of the work of Charlotte Selver and her husband, Charles V. W. Brooks, that "it cannot be described in words—it is the language of our spirit and being. They are among the greatest guides I know to the new or forgotten world in which mind and body are one." Between ancient Japan and modern Germany there is an immense cultural distance, which vanishes instantaneously when human somas become actively aware of themselves.

Aikido is a somatic discipline developed in Japan by Morihei Ueshiba during the close of the nineteenth century. It is not a system of combat or self-defense. It is, rather, a serene manner of playing with the forces involved in combat. Aikido is an active serenity that has its source in efficiency of movement and a simultaneous awareness of both oneself and one's "attacker." Confident in his coordination and balance, the trained practitioner of aikido greets the oncoming energy of his "attacker" and merges with it, never losing balance, control, or awareness. He throws his opponent in one smooth, impeccable motion or is himself thrown with the same efficient ease. As in Zen, the discipline is neither of "body" nor of "mind" but of the indissoluble unity of the human soma, and the adept holds himself balanced on the razor's edge where conscious intention and bodily movement become simultaneous and identical.

The Chinese tradition of Tai chi ch'uan is a somatic discipline similar to aikido, except that opponents and "throws" are not central. What is practiced is, essentially, a form of dance in which the individual goes through an exact choreography of balanced movements. Whereas aikido results in serenity and balance with the world, Tai chi ch'uan movements have an added theme: health. It is an ancient form of preventive medicine.

The most ancient of all disciplines in somatic education is yoga, a tradition that, like Zen, is incomprehensible from a Western religious point of view. The intention of yoga is the liberation and consolidation of one's self—"self" being conceived of, essentially, as a soma. The state of *samadhi* and the goal of *nirvritti* are not nonsomatic, "spiritual" goals but, instead, are attainments of somatic integrity whereby all conceptual illusions have been overcome and the nature of one's individual identity is clarified. The eight stages of raja yoga are graduated steps of awareness and control of progressively subtler somatic functions. At the eighth and final stage, the yogi has presumably gained final knowledge and control of all somatic functions, and this constitutes his liberation.

During the twentieth century there has been a steady growth of appreciation in Western culture of these Asian disciplines. To the degree that Europeans and Americans have developed insight into the somatic domain, they seem to have "discovered" the Asian traditions of somatic education. The implications of somatic education are enormous, and we would not expect anything but a slow, piecemeal acceptance of these implications.

A clinically successful form of somatic education that at first blush might not seem to be "body work" is biofeedback. In biofeedback we use an instrument to help us become aware of physiological events that otherwise are beneath the threshold of our consciousness. Something as simple as a mirror can be used as a biofeedback tool—as Matthias Alexander demonstrated. But we gain much more specific knowledge of our body with electronic devices that measure brain waves, muscle tension, skin temperature, or skin electrical potential.

When a person becomes aware of specific bodily processes, he can gain a measure of control over them. Migraine headaches, for example, are difficult to control by standard medical therapy; since the dilation of cranial arteries around the scalp has no known cause, there is no clear remedy. But biofeedback researchers have found that if a migraine sufferer has temperature monitors taped to his fingers, he can gradually learn to raise or lower the temperature of his hands. The temperature rises as his blood vessels dilate, bringing more blood to the hands. This diversion of blood to his extremities relieves the blood pressure in his central cranial arteries, preventing the migraine pain. Often after only a few training sessions, someone who has suffered severe migraines for years will learn to have complete control of the migraine pain.

This is education rather than therapy. Nothing is removed; instead, something is added: knowledge and control. Bodily processes that were beyond a person's awareness become, through biofeedback, controllable. Gaining control through becoming aware of one's bodily processes is a general theme of the somatic educators. They see that what medicine and physiology have believed to be uncontrollable, involuntary processes are not uncontrollable after all. For the somatic educators, conscious awareness of what was previously unconscious is the gateway to change. They tend to see consciousness not as an abstract "mind" but as a potent neurophysiological function for controlling the body.

INTELLIGENCE, SANITY, AND MOVEMENT

Jean Ayres and Marian Chace

In the United States there are many Sensory Integration Treatment Centers. The one where Jean Ayres can be found is located in Torrance, California. Here, in a large room with tall ceilings, small bodies are moving: There are young children in the room, which is crammed with things to play, ride, swing, bounce, rock, roll, and hang on. Ropes and cables hang from the ceiling, supporting hammock nets and various balancing boards. There is a trampoline that will send you soaring upward like a rocket. There is a barrel, padded on the inside, so that you can get in it and roll around the room. There are rope ladders you can climb on like a monkey. Over near the wall is a marvelous raised platform, one side of which is an inclined ramp; on top is a scooter board.

A child puts on a protective helmet, just like a racing driver, and mounts the ramp. There is a lady there who holds the scooter board while he lies down on his stomach. The board is pointed in the right direction, which is toward a bridge made of empty cardboard boxes. The young driver is aiming to scoot right under the bridge without hitting the boxes. Poised and ready, he is given the necessary nudge, and down the ramp he plummets, careening across the floor toward the bridge, under which he almost passes, until his elbow hits the corner of one of the boxes, whereupon the whole bridge comes tumbling down in grand confusion. Not only undaunted but absolutely delighted, he scrambles up and excitedly brings the scooter board back to the ramp, ready for another run.

He is playing. He and all the other children who are bouncing, balancing, climbing, and rolling are playing. And they are also doing something else: *They are becoming more intelligent.*

When he first started coming to this wonderful room, the young race driver could not lie on the scooter board and careen down the ramp. He did an odd thing: When lying on his stomach, his head drooped down over the edge of the board, almost touching the floor. For some reason he couldn't lift his head. When he clambered up on the huge ball, lying on his stomach, he could not help but cling to the ball, head down, hands and knees clutching the surface of the fabric. It felt very insecure up there.

Gradually with the aid of the net hammock and the ball and the balancing boards he began to lie down on his stomach and his head would lift up, so that he could see in front of him. His legs would also come up as the muscles in his back began to arch the whole of his body into a slight curve. Once he could move and balance and arch his body while lying on his stomach, he did the same thing on his hands and knees. At first it was frightening to lift his head up while balancing, like a young colt, simultaneously on four uncertain limbs. But bit by bit it became easier, it became fun. What had at first been scary became thrilling, just as the scooter board was thrilling when you tried to shift your weight to guide it under the bridge.

As he had more and more fun learning to do more and different things, his parents—and also his teacher—noticed that the restless, fidgety way in which he usually behaved was calming down. Before, he seemed to be always distracted, nervous; he could not sit still, nor could he fix his attention for long on anything. In school, he simply could not learn. Even the simplest tasks seemed beyond him, as if he was not organized to do them, not yet ready for school. Other children his age could perform the same tasks. He could not. He was not "normal." His parents began to hear such frightening terms as "brain damaged," "retarded," "learning disabled."

When his parents first took him to the big room in Torrance with all the things to play on, they met the woman who had devised all of these wonderful things. She had the lean face of a pioneer American woman, a frontier woman —which she most certainly is. She is Jean Ayres, who out of her concern for the many children who, at school age, are discovered to be abnormally developed, plunged into the task of making sense of the problem. Her plunge was straight into the jungle of neurophysiology and developmental psychology. She emerged from this jungle with an understanding of early human development that ranks her as one of the great American pioneers in what can be called somatic education.

Ayres' trail-blazing book *Sensory Integration and Learning Disorders* was her gift to the thousands of stunned parents who have discovered that their child has not developed normally. By virtue of her research, she began to see children as many-layered biological beings, whose "normalcy" is the composite coming together of ancient and primal functions that are not simply human, not simply simian, but extend through the quadrupedal functions of the higher vertebrates, down through the balancing functions of the fish, and back down to the primordial functions of the earliest somas. It is this same recognition of evolutionary functions that made possible the equally dramatic work with brain-damaged children developed at Philadelphia's Institutes for the Achievement of Human Potential by Temple Fay, Glenn Doman, and Carl Delacato.

Lying prone on a scooter board as it goes down a ramp is a way of stimulating one of these primordial functions: the standing function. During the first months of a child's life, the normal infant begins his mastery of the universal force of gravity. This mastery is the key to his survival. When the infant is placed on his stomach—the same position as his quadruped ancestors—he is automatically stimulated to do a most important thing: lift his head. He lifts his head against gravity, tensing the muscles in his neck and back and buttocks. This surprises parents, who at first cannot believe that an infant so young and weak would have either the inclination or the strength to lift such a large head.

The infant's action is not only an effort to use antigravity muscles but the attempt to raise the head to a horizontal position, so that the infant experiences what it feels like for the head to be balanced upward with the eyes looking forward at the line of the horizon. In this simple, primal, genetically programmed reflex the fledgling human being (1) makes his first movement upward; (2) directs his face forward; and (3) begins to relate his vision to the horizontal plane. He will persist in practicing this movement until, by five or six months, the entire musculature of the neck, back, and buttocks can lift head, arms, and legs off the floor in a lovely antigravity curve. He is learning the rudimentary stages of standing upright. Soon he will do the same thing on all fours and begin crawling. And, later, he will have the inner urge to stand up on two legs only.

All this learning is not merely "bodily" learning; rather, it is somatic learning. He is simultaneously learning "mental" abilities. It is exactly the same thing—so much so that if the development of the antigravity muscles is somehow disturbed, then the child's intelligence does not develop normally. So-called mental abilities *are* bodily abilities, but because we have for so long deluded ourselves that there is a "mind" that is different and separate from the "body," we have been incapable of seeing the obvious and ancient identity of the two.

In *Sensory Integration and Learning Disorders,* Jean Ayres gives us her theory in a nutshell:

> Essentially, the theory holds that disordered sensory integration accounts for some aspects of learning disorders and that enhancing sensory integration will make academic learning easier for those children whose problem lies in that domain. Sensory integration, or the ability to organize sensory information for use, can be improved through controlling its input to activate brain mechanisms (p. 1).

The hammocks and barrels and trampolines found in centers for Sensory Integration are the means for controlling the input of sensory information, giving specific sensations that the child is in need of experiencing. In the newborn baby two reflexes dominate its movements: the tonic labyrinthine reflex and the tonic neck reflex. The former (TLR) is directly stimulated by the force of gravity; it is a progravity reflex, which causes the infant to burrow its head downward, whether it is lying on its stomach or on its back. The TLR has the survival value of moving the neonate to burrow into the mother, clinging to her body. The latter reflex (TNR) is a fishlike swimming movement, stimulated by sense receptors in the neck joints. When the head is turned to the right, for example, the flexor muscles of the right arm contract, bringing the hand and shoulder up near the face; simultaneously, the extensor muscles on the left side contract, bringing the left arm down. If the head is moved left and right, the infant will, in effect, "swim," doing the Australian crawl.

These ancient reflexes that are present at birth will gradually fade away during the first months of development. Since they are progravity reflexes, they must be gradually inhibited by the higher learning centers of the cortex. The development of the antigravity muscles (the extensor muscles of the neck and back) is a process of learning to inhibit and control these reflexes that originate from lower and earlier centers of the brain. In most children the sensations of spontaneous movement and of being picked up, played with, held, and laid down are sufficient to stimulate the activation of the antigravity muscles. In some infants, this normal sensory stimulation is insufficient. Neither the TLR nor the TNR is inhibited, and the child is hunched forward insecurely, wanting to cling to gravity. In this situation, the child can no more master the up-down, left-right movements of vertical-horizontal space than he can master the movements involved in writing letters that go up and down, all the while following a horizontal line to the right, then dropping down to the next line and moving all the way back to the left-hand margin. Because reading involves these same movements by the eyes, the child cannot control the eye movement sufficiently to learn to read. Such a child has a learning disability, which is to say that his sensorimotor abilities have not developed at the rate one should expect. The functions of standing, facing, and handling have not yet been integrated by the timing function.

Inasmuch as the basic problem is that the antigravity muscles have not been stimulated into activity, special stimulation is needed. Some children need to have their developmental reflexes prodded, and that is precisely what is done at a center for Sensory Integration. Specific sensory stimulation is supplied that is strong and exciting enough to trigger an antigravity response. When the child careens down the ramp on his scooter board, the sudden thrilling drop downward and the acceleration of speed are fragments of sensory information that trigger a motor response: the lifting of the head and the arching of the back.

This is education—somatic education. It is something more primitive and fundamental than reading, writing, language skills, and all that acculturation teaches the child. The work of Jean Ayres informs us that the intellectual, "mental" attainments of "intelligence" are, at their core, the thatchwork of a prior, nonverbal learning of movement in the three dimensions of space, all coordinated in the proper temporal sequence. Without this layer of nonverbal, space-time learning there will be no intelligence. It is fascinating that our accomplishments in education and culture rest absolutely on a base of nonverbal, spatial-temporal abilities, which make these accomplishments possible. This primitive, somatic core of functions must be developed and integrated in order that the human being can learn how to learn.

Inasmuch as the child's mastery of the spatial-temporal realm takes place via the higher centers of the cortex, inhibiting reflexes in the lower centers of the brain, we should not be surprised if brain damage to the cortex would cause an adult to regress back to an infantile lack of antigravity reflexes. This is, in fact, what does happen either with accidental blows causing brain damage or with chronic schizophrenia.

Rehabilitation therapists at the Arizona State Hospital (King, 1974) had noticed the following somatic traits in those patients diagnosed as nonparanoid schizophrenics: (1) their posture showed, from the side, a pronounced head-to-toe S curve; (2) a shuffling gait; (3) inability to raise the arms above the head; (4) inability to rotate the head and great anxiety if the head was tilted backward (i.e., neck extension); (5) a tendency to hold the arms against the body (like a neonate infant) in a flexed, adducted position; and (6) a weakness and clumsiness in hand function. Although adults, they were, somatically, like children with a learning disability.

So it was decided to apply Jean Ayres' thinking to schizophrenic adults. The patients were invited to play noncompetitive games, such as tossing a balloon or ball back and forth, marching to music, stepping over ropes, ducking under the volleyball net, and so on. After two or three weeks, some very visible changes were noticed. The formerly sluggish, unmotivated, nonvocal patients were moving toward becoming the very opposite. Patients who had not spoken for years began to take part in conversations. There was greater attention paid to their personal appearance. They began to smile and become more mobile. The new sensory stimulation was having the same effect on these afflicted adults as it had on children with similar postural and movement limitations.

What the Arizona State Hospital discovered in the 1970s was what the staff of Saint Elizabeth's Hospital, in Washington, D.C., discovered in 1942 when Marian Chace created the profession of dance therapy. Chace, who was a modern dancer and teacher of dance, saw the withdrawn, incommunicable loneliness and silence of the psychotic patient. Intuitively, she knew that words were useless in bridging this gap. Movement was the answer.

> Basic dance is one of the most effective means to cut through this isolation, when the loneliness cannot be expressed and the preoccupation with this emotion is too intense to converse about other matters. Even when a lack of initiative prevents a patient from joining a group moving together in rhythm, the observation of such a group in rhythmic action may make a bond which will cut through the distance maintained by the patient. Basic dance is the externalization of those inner feelings which can only be shared in rhythmic, symbolic action (Chaiklin, 1975, p. 170).

During her twenty years at Saint Elizabeth's, Chace's work came to be considered an irreplaceable part of the total rehabilitative program of the hospital. As her success came to be better known, the dance therapy movement began to grow. In every instance its developers were dancers whose teaching later developed into therapy. All of these early developers were modern dancers: Franziska Boas and Lilyan Espenak on the East Coast, and Trudi Schoop and Mary Whitehouse on the West Coast. They had, as modern dancers, broken away from the formal theatricality of classical ballet to plunge into a new world of elemental, expressive movements. It was this radically different attitude toward movement that characterized modern dance and predisposed it to see all human movement as expressive of the mental-emotional nature of the human. For the psychotically withdrawn, movement was the needed vehicle for expression and renewed contact with others and with the world.

For afflicted children and adults, it is movement and the sensations of movement that chart the pathway to a focused consciousness and an effective life. For too many years therapists had been intoxicated with words and with the illusions of what words can do. In basic situations such as the learning-disabled child or the schizophrenic adult, words are powerless. The problem lies at another, more fundamental level: the wordless sensations of vertical and horizontal movements integrated in temporal sequence. It is this primordial, somatic level that makes all speech and all language possible.

Jean Ayres and Marian Chace (as well as Fay, Doman, and Delacato) saw the crucial significance of this nonverbal realm and discovered how to gain access to it. Both women reached past the maya of words and seized hold of the silent core of the human being, a creature who, before all else, feels and moves.

INTEGRATING NEURAL FUNCTIONS

Moshe Feldenkrais

Moshe Feldenkrais is a man full of surprises. He is one of the world's great authorities on human sensorimotor functions, but at the same time he is a research physicist who spent many years side by side with the Nobel laureate Frédéric Joliot-Curie, doing nuclear fission work in Paris. He built the Van de Graaff nuclear accelerator, which still awes Parisian schoolchildren when they visit the Petit Palais d'Exposition, but he also was Europe's first black-belt judoka and founded the famous Jiu-Jitsu Club de France.

When he was chased from France by the Nazi invasion, his talents were put to use by the British admiralty in the development of radar for antisubmarine warfare; but at the same time, he became fascinated with the thinking of the Russian philosopher Gurdjieff and the body posture work of F. Matthias Alexander. After the war, he returned to Israel's Ministry of Defense, Electronics Division, but he surprised everyone by dropping his electronics work and going full-time into working with human neuromuscular problems.

In 1973 I had come to Berkeley, California, to spend one month learning Feldenkrais' Awareness Through Movement exercises. These exercises are ingenious and gentle ways of integrating new sensorimotor patterns into our central nervous system. The changes in the range and quality of movement are extraordinary. That in itself was already a revelation to me, for it confirmed that Feldenkrais was one of the practical experts in the somatic field. In 1969 I had written *Bodies in Revolt: A Primer in Somatic Thinking,* the first general survey of the field. In 1971 I had spent a year studying neurophysiology at the University of Florida Medical School, after which I was beginning to think that everyone was content to divide the human being into the religious schism of "body" and "mind" but that no one was concerned to have a unitary scientific conception of the living human being. Having heard of Feldenkrais (the last syllable rhymes with *rice*), I read one of his works, *Body and Mature Behavior,* and sought him out in Berkeley during one of his rare visits to the United States.

During the third week of the movement exercises, the class had a visitor. It was a man who had known of Feldenkrais and had flown to Berkeley from Washington, D.C. His name was George, and he was a classic instance of the terrible damage cerebral palsy can wreak on a person, a disease with which he had been stricken at three years of age. Now fifty-three years old, George's body was folded in upon itself from the middle line—arms and legs turned inward as he moved, his whole body an uncoordinated cascade of spastic heaves and jerks, face contorted, and with a voice that sounded like a barking seal. Even his breathing was uncoordinated and jerky; his chest percolated with a spasmodic panting. I had no idea why he was there or what help he could expect. It was obvious that he could not do the exercises; he had too little control of his body movements.

Feldenkrais stopped the class, cleared a space, and set up a long, narrow table, just big enough to lie down on. He laid a blanket on it, found a small roller to use as a head rest, and asked George to lie down. Lying on the table, George was anything but tranquil. Involuntarily, his chest and stomach twitched arhythmically as he gasped for breath.

Feldenkrais leaned over and told him to be as passive as he possibly could and to try not to do anything at all. Then Feldenkrais brought his hands down to George's chest and began to press the rib cage, very slowly and gently. He would change his position and put pressures in different directions through the rib cage, occasionally going down to the abdominal muscles just underneath the bottom edge of the chest. He continued this for about twenty minutes, working intensely and saying nothing. Toward the end of this time, he would press the lower edge of the chest and hold it for a long moment and then release it, hold it again and then release it. He did this, reminding George not to help, not to do anything.

At a certain instant, something uncanny happened: George seemed to become quieter. His chest was no longer heaving spasmodically. Feldenkrais continued to press, hold, and release, occasionally changing the angle of pressure slightly. Then he released the chest a final time and stepped back. George lay there, serenely breathing in a quiet, slow, rhythmical pattern. His face showed his astonishment. He could not believe what was happening. Nor could I. I realized that my cheeks were wet. Fifty years of fitful, nightmarish breathing had vanished in twenty minutes. Fifty years of presumably deeply enrooted habit, impossible to eradicate, disappeared in a few minutes. And how? *By one human being helping another human being move in a certain way.*

I had just witnessed my first demonstration of Functional Integration. Despite my bewilderment, I had not seen a "miracle," nor had I seen a "healing" or a "cure." I had seen what Feldenkrais modestly described as a "lesson." He had "taught" George to breathe normally.

But he wasn't done. With George now lying there, face flushed and eyes shining above the gently rising and falling chest, Feldenkrais took hold of his right hand. The fingers were not really fingers; they were a spastic knot—all four were as if bound together into a constricted curve. They were not four fingers but one. Feldenkrais began tickling the little finger, teasing it and helping it, apparently, to become even more spastic. But that is not what happened. What happened was that after a few minutes the little finger began to shiver and then tremble. *It began to move independently.*

He then left the hand and went up to George's face. He asked George to open his mouth and stick his tongue out and then to move it to the left and to the right. While George did that, Feldenkrais pressed underneath the chin and moved the jaw slightly. At first, George could not control his tongue and jaw movements very well, but soon, by doing these tiny movements, the control became more precise. He asked George to say something. When the words came out, they no longer sounded like those of a barking seal. A change had taken place: There was greater clarity.

Then Feldenkrais stopped. Thirty minutes had gone by, and George was now breathing normally, differentiating the movement of his right little finger, and gaining control of his speech for the first time in fifty years. And all by the simple use of hands. The somatic terrain had suddenly been revealed to me in a quick, precise manner by a seventy-year-old man who had already explored that territory and mapped out a mighty portion of the terrain. He was no faith healer. Indeed, as a scientist with a positivistic bent, he had absolute scorn and disbelief for such claims. He was quite simply a scientist who had extended his knowledge about the world of physics into the functions of the human soma. He knew about gravity, he knew about the mechanics of movement, and he knew about the cybernetics of coordination in a self-correcting, living system. At that moment I made a decision: I would learn to do Functional Integration.

Which I did. I had the good fortune to be in charge of a graduate school in San Francisco, and Feldenkrais accepted my invitation to become a Distinguished Visiting Professor for a three-year period, teaching the theory and techniques of Functional Integration. Some sixty people from various parts of the world enrolled in the course, and during three successive summers they gathered in San Francisco to study with Feldenkrais. In the interims between the summers they practiced what they had learned.

From the beginning it was clear that this was to be an

unusual course of study. On the first day Feldenkrais announced the basic principle of Functional Integration: "The first principle of my work is that there isn't any principle." The first third of the course was a gradual deprogramming of the usual ways in which most people think about "bodies." When one looks at another person's "body," one must realize that he is observing the moving process of that person's "mind." When someone thinks and experiences, he does so through "bodily" movement; the human being cannot think without moving. Feldenkrais illustrates this point by inviting anyone "mentally" to count from one to ten as fast as he can and then to try doubling that speed. Abruptly one realizes there is an absolute limit to the speed with which one can count. If counting were purely "mental," quite separate from "bodily" processes, there would be no limit to how fast one could count. But as soon as one attempts to exceed a certain limit, one realizes that one is using quick subverbal movements and that one can go from one number to the next only as quickly as one can make these movements. The crucial point is that all human conscious and unconscious experience is physiological: It is organic movement.

But as this conceptual deprogramming proceeded, it was replaced by something else, a gradually cultivated awareness of one's self as a balancing, moving, integrating being. Understanding another human being is not, first of all, a conceptual task but a perceptual task. One must learn to see all that is happening with another person. Without training one's ability to sense the raw, nonverbal expressions of life, one lacks the essential equipment for interpreting another person's behavior. Thus it was as simple as this: In order to be maximally sensitive to another person, one must be maximally sensitive to oneself.

This is something that everyone, in the inner sanctum of his thoughts, already knows. How can anyone understand and help another if he has not already attained some ability to understand and help himself? This is so obvious as to be beyond question, yet when we look at the training systems in medicine and psychotherapy, we find almost a complete absence of this concern. Instead, one is taught information and one is taught techniques, and these are the conceptual and practical tools that the therapist uses to "help" his patient.

One cannot receive health from the sick; one cannot receive balance from the imbalanced; one cannot be understood by someone who cannot understand himself, nor can one be helped by someone who cannot help himself —this is a hard dictum and an obvious one. Even so, it is all but nonexistent in the training programs of the health-related professions.

So the pedagogy of Moshe Feldenkrais was to replace conceptual attitudes with perceptual abilities. This is why the first principle of his work is that there is no principle. Learning to appreciate Functional Integration is, initially, learning to appreciate yourself. First work on yourself, then work on others. And this is the way things proceeded. What was fascinating was that to the degree that one became aware of one's own internal kinesthetic and proprioceptive senses, one became more aware of the same thing in others.

The second stage was learning to touch other people and move their bodies. It quickly became apparent that one can understand and diagnose the general state of another human being simply by touching and moving that person's limbs—*if* one is maximally sensitive to the quality of the movement. When, for instance, another person is lying down on his back and is instructed to be passive and make no voluntary movement, we might think that his body would be relaxed, supple, and easy to move. This is not the case. *When passive, every human body responds differently to movement.* What one discovers is that beneath the level of conscious, voluntary movement, every individual has an unconscious program of involuntary movement. One of the first virtues of Functional Integration is that *it makes the individual aware of his or her unconscious patterns of habitual behavior.* The man who is anxious all the time displays a body that is anxious all the time. The woman who is chronically angry has a body that is chronically angry. The child who is constantly afraid has a muscular system that is always tensed in fright. The widow who is depressed has a physiological system that is, in every respect, depressed.

If you place your hand on the forehead of a person lying on his back and gently rotate the head a little to the left and right, the quality of that movement tells you of the general state of that person. If you, one by one, rotate the heads of one hundred different persons, you will feel a different quality of movement in each one. The different ways in which heads move testify to the different ways in which each person habitually uses and experiences his neck, his chest, and his entire trunk. The head of one person will move back and forth relatively easily, except that in one place there will be a "sticky" spot where the muscles seize and hold the head. In another person the head may be so rigidly fixated that it will hardly move, even though the person is not voluntarily holding it stiffly.

In another person the head may move freely to the right and hardly move at all to the left, as is often the case with people who have torticollis, or wryneck. When their heads are rotated, some people unconsciously "help" the movement; the instant they sense that you are moving the head to the left, they cannot prevent taking control and helpfully moving it to the left. Often women who from childhood have been cowed into obedient cooperation cannot stop helpfully accommodating themselves to any direction of movement suggested; they are habituated to being manipulated. As soon as they, as adults, *become aware* of this heretofore unconscious habituation, they have made the first step in dehabituating this internal tyranny.

The qualities of unconscious movement in the human body are as individual as one's personality or character structure, because *these habitual patterns of acting are the somatic structure of what we call personality and character.* When I feel specific patterns of habituated movements in a human being, I am not feeling that person's "body"; rather, I am feeling that person as that person is habitually structured to act, to think, and to experience himself. Functional Integration does not have to do with "bodies"; it has to do with the entire living individual. The anxiety, fear, anger, or depression that I can feel in a person is exactly the same anxiety, fear, anger, or depression that that person feels and experiences as the constant undertone of his own existence.

We do not fear without muscles and sinew that fear. We cannot hate or be angry without an organism that hates and is angry. We cannot love and hope and expect without actively, movingly, physiologically loving and hoping and expecting. Hate, anger, love, and hope are not "psychological states" existing in some "mental" vacuum; they are *somatic* states that exist in the entirety of our living system.

But wait. If these are somatic states, palpably observable within our flesh, then to change these habitual patterns of action is to change these states. If the neuromuscular system of a widow is depressed, then if she is taught to change that pattern, she will no longer be depressed.

Functional Integration is a method of *somatic education.* As such, the improvements that come about are just as "psychological" as they are "physiological." They are systemic, affecting the entire living organism. The system that is affected is the four-dimensional process by which the human being organizes his actions in this very real world of length, depth, width, and time. With two hands one can feel how the individual has learned to use the vertical, horizontal, and temporal patterns of movement that are his primordial functions. And because they have been learned during the course of that person's lifetime, *they can be unlearned and replaced with new learning.*

Somatic education involves the systemic change of the entire human being. The personality, the direction, the intentions of the person are modified. The human process is modified so that the individual proceeds through time in a different way. Because he is a physicist, Feldenkrais implicitly understands the gravitational and structural lines of force with which the human must contend as he makes his way through this world. In the same way, he understands that the human soma is a neurally organized cybernetic system that is self-adjusting, self-correcting, and self-improving—*if* that system is given new information with which to interact and *if* that system is allowed to become *sensorily aware* that there are other options than the ways in which it habitually acts. The human soma is self-improving because it has an ancient, built-in bias toward efficiency.

In his teaching, Moshe Feldenkrais made sure that his students first became more sensorily aware of themselves, so that, secondarily, they could be maximally aware of the quality of movement in others. With that learned, the third stage for the Functional Integrationist was to learn the various systemic movements one could introduce into the human being so as to teach new patterns of movement. These various systemic movements are as fundamentally somatic as all the rest of Functional Integration: They follow the principles of physical mechanics, kinesiology, and neurophysiology.

For many years Feldenkrais has worked with his friend Peter Brook, the theatrical director, who lives alternately in England and in France. In London and in Paris Feldenkrais teaches actors how to improve their expressive movements and to expand the range of their movements. In the same cities he will leave the theater and go to a hospital to give a demonstration of how spastic paralysis can be overcome by teaching movement to the victim.

What Functional Integration accomplishes is, from the viewpoint of traditional medicine, impossible. It is extremely difficult for physicians to accept the fact that ailments that are untreatable medically can be made to disappear by nonmedical procedures. Laypersons have the same difficulty, because they, too, have been taught to think about the human body in terms of the medical model. In both cases, the disbelief is based on an implicit pessimism that claims that certain functions of human beings are unchangeable. As it turns out, physicians and their patients both accept functional disorders as inevitable and as the effects of old age or unknown causes. "You'll just have to learn to live with it" are the accepted words of advice.

It was this same pessimism that was encountered by the two great developers of biofeedback technology, Joe Kamiya and Barbara Brown. No one believed that autonomic, involuntary functions could be controlled by the individual. It could not be believed, even though this was precisely what was being done and reported over and over again in consistent, predictable fashion by biofeedback laboratories.

Somatic education is not only something new and unexpected, it is something of momentous consequence: It entails a basic transformation in our understanding of the human species and of the capacities of the human individual. That which we have believed to be unchangeable in the human creature has been discovered to be not, after all, so unchangeable. Such a discovery amounts to a reassessment of the nature of ourselves and of humankind.

It is inevitable that the procedures of Functional Integration and biofeedback will become accepted as indispensable adjuncts to a newly envisioned system of medicine. I believe that it is also inevitable that the gentle transformatory effects of Awareness Through Movement exercises will become a permanent part of the physical-mental educational programs made available to both schoolchildren and adults. Used in school systems, these exercises will not only help children to grow better balanced and coordinated but will save them from the proprioceptive apathy that is the chief killer of functionally distorted adults. If physical-education curricula were expanded to include regular experiences of Awareness Through Movement, we would discover, one generation later, that the major diseases of public health—the functionally caused diseases—were fast disappearing.

Moshe Feldenkrais is one of the great benefactors of mankind, and the benefits he has bestowed are only now coming to be discovered and appreciated. He himself is modest about what he does. He once said, "In the early days, when I had the notion that I was trying to 'cure' my client, I did rather poor work. But later, when I realized the two of us were, in fact, working together to achieve an understanding of the situation, then my work changed. Only then did it become more certain."

THREE / THE ARCHESOMA

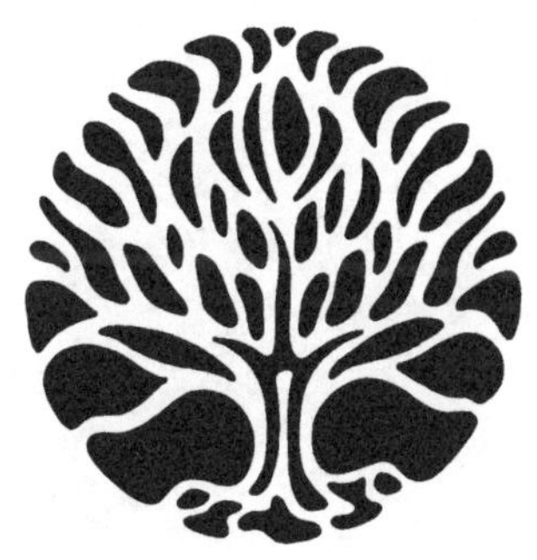

Functional Integration is, like other forms of somatic education, a practice that is in advance of its theory. We know the conditions under which Functional Integration is effective, but we do not necessarily know all the reasons why this should be the case. Despite the case histories and despite the discussion of somatic education, most readers may have the feeling that there is a central question yet to be answered: How does it work? What are the leading principles or practices of Functional Integration that bring about such changes in human beings? Or, put differently, what is it about human beings that makes the techniques of somatic education effective?

The answer to this is, of course, theoretical, but it is a theory with massive evidential support from research science as well as from somatic practitioners. The main body of the answer has been developed in the course of this book. It is the theory of the archesoma, which holds that because all life involves movement, every living creature has in its constitution a simple core of movement possibilities defined by the three dimensions of space and the dimension of time. The archesoma is a basic system of movements possessed in common by all species of creatures, undergirding their behavior and determining the efficiency of their actions.

Because the body of life was, from its formation, an integrated system of movement, it was a four-dimensional entity whose first law was efficiency. The evolution of life has been dominated by this efficiency principle, which selects for survival those structures and functions that improve efficiency and, therefore, adaptation.

The archesoma is just as powerfully present in human beings as in any other species, and is at the core of human functioning, just as the hub is at the center of the wheel. All human functions—physiological, psychological, emotional, and so forth—are direct reflections of the state of the archesoma, which operates at the core of these functions, rendering them either more effective and coordinated or less so. The archesoma is the general precondition for all specific movements: If the core is distorted, so will the specific physiological, psychological, perceptual, judgmental, and all other functions be distorted and less effective.

It is also important to remember that this primitive aspect of neural functioning occupies center stage in the human sensorimotor system, the neural system that lies at the structural-functional heart of the central nervous system. Thus the condition of the archesoma is objectively observable by its patterns of movements and subjectively observable by the proprioceptive sensations of these movement patterns. These archesomatic patterns are nonverbal; they lie just beneath the verbal acculturation that is constructed on top of the archesoma. As we know from Jean Ayres, if the archesomatic functions are poorly developed, the perceptual and intellectual functions will also be poorly developed. What we call the mind emerges from the archesomatic core and is no more nor less efficient than this core is. Also, we know from Marian Chace that the mental and emotional life is so directly reflective of the archesomatic process that if we improve this process, the mental and emotional functions improve.

The various forms of somatic education all assume that the archesoma can learn and that any improvement in movement will be an improvement in all human functioning. Keep in mind that archesomatic learning is general. It does not involve learning a special skill but, rather, prepares us for learning and executing a special skill. Learning to play golf or handball is, for example, a special skill for a special purpose, but the level of efficiency of the skill directly depends on the efficiency of the archesoma. It provides the repertory of range, coordination, and balance of sensorimotor functions that are used in the learning of golf or handball. No matter how hard one works to improve one's golfing skill, the final determinant of improvement will be the archesoma. If one's internal sensing and control is faulty, then one's ability to perform any skill is hampered. We can learn how to do any particular skill, but the efficiency level of how we do it is dependent on the state of the functions of standing, facing, handling, and their integration through timing.

The nonverbal activities of the archesoma are not only

beneath the "mind" and the skills it learns, they also, for the same reason, escape the attention of the mind. The nonverbal realm of self-sensing is not at all in the forefront of consciousness; rather, it is in the background. It is normally unconscious. In adults whose proprioceptive senses have atrophied, the workings of the archesoma seem to be nonexistent. There is a schism between the conscious functions and the archesomatic functions. When this occurs, the archesoma, unobserved and unguided, can become distorted and inefficient, thus distorting the entire human system, rendering the human being clumsy and uncomfortable. When such an event occurs, it is of little use to address the psychological functions or the physiological structure; what is required is an improvement in the archesoma. This can take place only by becoming aware of the archesomatic functions and gaining greater range, coordination, and balance of these basic movements.

When the archesoma goes awry, distorting the ways in which we think, act, and react, these distortions are experienced as involuntary. The physiological, emotional, and psychological malfunctions happen automatically, without any awareness of their taking place nor with any conscious intention to do so. The art of Functional Integration involves detecting these involuntary, unconscious movements and making them voluntary and conscious again. For people whose self-sensing abilities are atrophied, the archesoma is almost synonymous with the unconscious, as if it were a biologically separate world. Yet if one's self-sensing abilities can be improved, the functions of the archesoma become both conscious and controllable.

How does Functional Integration do this? First, by creating the conditions for maximal awareness, namely, by allowing the body and the central nervous system to become quiescent. This is usually accomplished by having the person remove his nervous system from a vertical relation with gravity by lying horizontal on a comfortable surface. When one is lying horizontal, most voluntary movement is suspended. Consequently, if the practitioner moves some section of this recumbent body and notices muscular holdings and jerkiness, he can be sure that he has discovered the involuntary and unconscious activities of the archesoma.

The Functional Integrationist then serves as a midwife in the birth of new awareness and new voluntary control. He creates the conditions for discovering involuntary movements, and when he does so, both he and his client simultaneously become conscious of these movements. The client is always surprised: "I had no idea that my shoulders were so jerky and my spine so stiff." Once both client and practitioner are aware of the distorted, involuntary movements of the archesoma, they can turn to the task of learning greater sensorimotor control of these functions.

The many techniques by which Functional Integrationists teach improved sensorimotor function are centered on the effort to make the client fully aware of movements that he had forgotten or else had never learned. The practitioner becomes, as it were, the motor system of the client, moving the limbs and muscles through patterns that the client will never, of his own volition, be able to perform. By deliberately doing the work of the motor system for the client, he makes it possible for the client's sensory system to receive stimuli from the motor system that it otherwise never experiences. This new sensory information immediately serves as a guide for performing new motor patterns on the voluntary level. The goal of Functional Integration is to integrate the human being by integrating his sensorimotor functions.

There may be no creature other than the human being that can direct its awareness inwardly to its own bodily movements. Functional Integration and all forms of somatic education use this human ability to enlarge and improve the degree of our somatic self-awareness. Like two knitting needles, the sensory system and motor system are made to intertwine, creating a greater sensory awareness of our internal activities and a greater activity of our internal sensory awareness. The gain is in active self-awareness, and the realm of somatic education has made it certain that human awareness must be recognized as a biological force that can be as potent for human growth as it can be for human degeneration.

reading references

There are many forms of body therapy and body change other than those mentioned in this book and in this list of reading references. Therapists can work with the body or on the body in ways that are not identifiably somatic. Hence, this list includes only references that are specifically illustrative of functional, somatic concerns and not of the general bodily concerns of more traditional medicine and psychotherapy.

Alexander, F. Matthias. *The Resurrection of the Body.* New York: Delta, 1969.

Ayres, A. Jean. "Occupational Therapy Directed Toward Neuromuscular Integration." In *Occupational Therapy,* edited by H. S. Willard and C. S. Spackman. 3rd ed., rev. Philadelphia: J. B. Lippincott Co., 1963.

———. *Sensory Integration and Learning Disorders.* Los Angeles: Western Psychological Services, 1972.

Barlow, Wilfred. *The Alexander Technique.* Rochester, Vt.: Healing Arts Press, 1990.

Bartal, Lea, and Mira Ne'eman. *Movement Awareness and Creativity.* New York: Harper and Row, 1975.

Bertherat, Thérèse, and Carol Bernstein. *The Body Has Its Reasons.* Rochester, Vt.: Healing Arts Press, 1989.

Bogen, Joseph E. "The Other Side of the Brain I: Dysgraphia and Dyscopia Following Cerebral Commissurotomy." *Bulletin of the Los Angeles Neurological Societies* 34 (1969); 73–105.

——. "The Other Side of the Brain II: An Appositional Mind." *Bulletin of the Los Angeles Neurological Societies* 34 (1969): 13–62.

Bogen, Joseph E., and Glenda M. Bogen. "The Other Side of the Brain III: The Corpus Callosum and Creativity." *Bulletin of the Los Angeles Neurological Societies* 34 (1969): 191–220.

Brooks, Charles V. W. *Sensory Awareness: The Rediscovery of Experiencing.* New York: Harper and Row, 1974.

Brown, Barbara. *New Mind, New Body.* New York: Harper and Row, 1975.

——. *Stress and the Art of Biofeedback.* New York: Harper and Row, 1977.

Chaiklin, Harris, ed. *Marian Chace: Her Papers.* New York: American Dance Therapy Association, 1975.

Costonis, Maureen N., ed. *Therapy in Motion.* Urbana, Ill.: University of Illinois Press, 1978.

Darwin, Charles. *The Expression of the Emotions in Man and Animals.* Chicago: University of Chicago Press, 1965.

Davis, Roland C. "Patterns of Muscular Activity During 'Mental Work' and Their Constancy." *Journal of Experimental Psychology* 24 (1939): 451–65.

Delacato, Carl H. *The Treatment and Prevention of Reading Problems: The Neuro-Psychological Approach.* Springfield, Ill.: Charles C. Thomas, 1959.

——. *Neurological Organization and Reading.* Springfield, Ill.: Charles C. Thomas, 1966.

Eibl-Eibesfeldt, Irenaus. *Ethology: The Biology of Behavior.* New York: Holt, Rinehart and Winston, 1970.

Feldenkrais, Moshe. *Judo.* London: Frederick Warne, 1942.

——. *Higher Judo.* 3 vols. London: Frederick Warne, 1942.

——. *Body and Mature Behavior.* New York: International Universities Press, 1950.

——. *Awareness Through Movement.* New York: Harper and Row, 1972.

——. *Adventures in the Jungle of the Brain: The Case of Nora.* New York: Harper and Row, 1977.

Gardner, Martin. *The Ambidextrous Universe: Left, Right and the Fall of Parity.* New York: Mentor Books, 1964.

Hanna, Thomas. "The Living Body: Nexus of Process Philosophy and Existential Phenomenology." *Soundings* 52, no. 3 (Fall 1969): 323–33.

——. *Bodies in Revolt: A Primer in Somatic Thinking.* New York: Holt, Rinehart and Winston, 1970.

——. "The Project of Somatology." *Journal of Humanistic Psychology* 13, no. 3 (Summer 1973): 3–14.

——. "Three Elements of Somatology." *Main Currents in Modern Thought* 31, no. 3 (January–February 1975): 82–87.

——. "The Field of Somatics." *Somatics 1,* no. 1 (Autumn 1976): 30–34.

——. "The Somatic Healers and the Somatic Educators." *Somatics 1,* no. 3 (Autumn 1977): 48–52.

——, ed. *Explorers of Humankind.* San Francisco: Harper and Row, 1979.

Jacobson, E. *Progressive Relaxation.* 2d ed. Chicago: University of Chicago Press, 1938.

——. *Modern Treatment of Tense Patients.* Springfield, Ill.: Charles C. Thomas, 1970.

King, Lorna Jean. "A Sensory-Integrative Approach to Schizophrenia." *The American Journal of Occupational Therapy* 28, no. 9 (October 1974): 529–36.

Lorenz, Konrad. "The Evolution of Behavior." *Scientific American* 199, no. 6 (1958): 67–78.

——. *On Aggression.* New York: Harcourt, Brace and World, 1963.

Luce, Gay Gaer. *Biological Rhythms in Psychiatry and Medicine.* Washington, D. C.: National Institute of Mental Health, 1970.

——. *Body Time: Physiological Rhythms and Social Stress.* New York: Pantheon Books, 1971.

McGuigan, F. J. "Covert Oral Behavior During the Silent Performance of Language Tasks." *Psychological Bulletin* 74 (1970): 309–26.

Malmo, Robert B. *On Emotions, Needs, and Our Archaic Brain.* New York: Holt, Rinehart and Winston, Inc., 1975.

Monod, Jacques. *Chance and Necessity.* New York: Alfred A. Knopf, 1972.

Penfield, W., and L. Roberts. *Speech and Brain-Mechanisms.* Princeton, N. J.: Princeton University Press, 1959.

Pribram, Karl. "Human Consciousness and the Functions of the Brain," *Somatics* 1, no. 2 (Spring 1977): 5–70.

——. *Languages of the Brain: Experimental Paradoxes and Principles in Neuropsychology.* Englewood Cliffs, N.J.: Prentice-Hall, 1971.

Schoop, Trudi. *Won't You Join the Dance?* Palo Alto, Calif.: Mayfield Publishing Company, 1974.

Selye, Hans. *The Stress of Life.* New York: McGraw-Hill Book Co., 1956.

——. *Stress Without Distress.* New York: J. B. Lippincott Co., 1974.

Sherrington, Charles. *The Integrative Action of the Nervous System.* New Haven: Yale University Press, 1906.

——. *Man on His Nature.* Garden City, N.Y.: Doubleday and Co., 1940.

Smith, S. M., H. O. Brown, J. E. P. Toman, and L. S. Goodman. "The Lack of Cerebral Effects of d-tubocuranine." *Anesthesiology* 8 (1947): 1–14.

Sperry, Roger W. "Neurology and the Mind-Brain Problem." *American Scientist* 40 (1952): 291–312.

——. "Physiological Plasticity and Brain Circuit Theory." In *Biological and Biochemical Bases of Behavior,* edited by H. F. Harlow and C. N. Woolsey. Madison: University of Wisconsin Press, 1958.

——. "Some Developments in Brain Lesion Studies of Learning." Federation Proceedings 20, pt. 1 (1961): 601–16.

Sperry, Roger W., and Michael S. Gazzaniga. "Language Following Surgical Disconnection of the Hemispheres." In *Brain Mechanisms Underlying Speech and Language,* edited by C. H. Millikan and F. L. Darley. New York: Grune and Stratton, 1967.

Wallerstein, H. "An Electromyographic Study of Attentive Listening." *Canadian Journal of Psychology* 8 (1954): 228–38.

Wittrock, M. C. ed. *The Human Brain.* Englewood Cliffs, N. J.: Prentice-Hall, 1977.

N.B. As a general source of information on the somatic field, see *Somatics: Magazine-Journal of the Bodily Arts and Sciences,* 1516 Grant Ave., Suite 220, Novato, California 94947.

index

Note: **Bold** page numbers refer to illustrations and figures